FORKED

A New Standard for American Dining

Saru Jayaraman

OXFORD
UNIVERSITY PRESS

OXFORD
UNIVERSITY PRESS

Oxford University Press is a department of the University of Oxford. It furthers the University's objective of excellence in research, scholarship, and education by publishing worldwide.Oxford is a registered trade mark of Oxford University Press in the UK and certain other countries.

Published in the United States of America by Oxford University Press
198 Madison Avenue, New York, NY 10016, United States of America.

© Saru Jayaraman 2016

First Edition published in 2016

Cataloging-in-Publication data is on file at the Library of Congress
ISBN 978-0-19-938047-3

1 3 5 7 9 8 6 4 2

Printed by Sheridan, USA

To the 11 million restaurant workers nationwide.

To my children, who say they want to be
'ROC star' restaurant workers when they grow up.

And to everyone who works to make this
industry better for all of us.

CONTENTS

ACKNOWLEDGMENTS

This book was most definitely a team effort. First, many thanks to everyone at ROC: our amazing restaurant worker members and leaders; the many fabulous restaurant employer members who partner with Restaurant Opportunities Center (ROC), many of whom are profiled in this book; board members of Diners United, the new and growing group of consumers who are paving the way for a new kind of consumer movement; our donors and funders, especially the Ford Foundation for helping to launch this book; and our board, allies, executive team, and staff all over the country. For research assistance, connections to subjects, and general support, many thanks to Christina Fletes, Teofilo Reyes, Mike Rodriguez, Michaela Allen, Graham Kovich, ROC Michigan members, Dania Rajendra, Alex Galimberti, Lauren Jacobs, Kennard Ray, and professors and students at the University of California, Berkeley, the University of North Carolina at Chapel Hill, and the University of Georgia. For fabulous and creative thinking around the book and getting the word out, many thanks to Ariel Jacobson, Maria Myotte, and Elspeth Gilmore, and ROC's filmmaker and creative genius

Sekou Luke. Last but not least, many thanks to my co-founders and co-conspirators Fekkak Mamdouh and Sekou Siby.

Thanks to Oxford editor Chad Zimmerman for his faith and support throughout the process, to my agent Regina Brooks, and to my family. Thanks to my parents, sisters, and nephews for their constant love and support. To Zach, Akeela, and Lina, thank you for making everything possible!

[1]

INTRODUCTION

Why We Are Forked

People know me as the co-founder and co-director of the Restaurant Opportunities Centers (ROC) United, a national social-movement organization dedicated to raising wages and working conditions in the nation's restaurant industry. I have dedicated my life to serving as an organizer, advocate, and spokesperson for raising standards for restaurant workers.

What almost no one knows about me is that I don't come from a line of restaurant *workers*; I come from a family of restaurant *owners*. And the family restaurant did not pay its workers well.

In the early 1900s, my great-great grandfather, a policeman named Sundara, opened a large restaurant in the tiny town of Karur, India. Motivated in part by his disdain for working for others (a sentiment shared today by his descendant), Sundara decided to open his own place, and call it Sundara Villas. Since the proprietor was an Indian Brahmin, Sundara Villas was forbidden by caste from serving meat. The cuisine was South Indian vegetarian, served communal-style on washed banana leaves to guests seated at long marble tables.

In those days, the general rule—and preference—was to eat at home, specifically a meal cooked by a wife or mother. Men only ate

1

in restaurants if they were traveling, or a bachelor, or if their wives were sick or traveling. Gender norms forbade women from eating out or mixing with men in such public spaces, and thus the restaurant was almost an entirely male affair, with the exception of the proprietor's daughters and granddaughters, who would run around playing in the restaurant.

Sundara brought his sons to work in the restaurant, but also hired young men from Karur and the neighboring villages. These workers were paid meager monthly wages, and many slept in the restaurant itself.

My great-grandfather, Venkataramanaswamy (try that ten times!), took over the restaurant when Sundara died. He also brought his sons to work in the restaurant. At this point there were young men who had worked at the restaurant for a lifetime, literally. And although wages were meager, there was most definitely a sense of family. Workers who fell ill were neither asked to work nor docked pay. Servers and cooks became lifelong family members. The longest-lasting server, a man named Sundaram, volunteered to cook at my parents' wedding and attended every family wedding and function after that; my great-grandfather paid for Sundaram's son's coming-of-age ceremony. Another cook worked both in the restaurant and in the house, washing the children's clothes.

There is no way I could call my great-grandfather a "high road" employer, which is the label we at ROC give to employers who provide their employees with livable wages and working conditions. The sense of family that my parents used to describe the restaurant is the same word almost every restaurateur in America uses to describe their employees—generally without cause and as a justification for paying low wages. We at ROC always respond by saying that being a family, although wonderful, is not enough; a family that keeps some of its relatives in poverty is a family that can do better, both for the sake of the workers and ultimately for the benefit of employers and consumers.

My restaurant-owning grandfathers were small business owners who followed the norms, customs, and culture of their day; today, these surrounding factors have changed and evolved. One hundred years later, their granddaughter is leading a movement to improve wages and working conditions for the workers they employed.

I love and respect my great-grandfather. He was a kind and extremely generous man who took care of his large family, his brothers' families, and even the families of his employees. Certainly, through his eyes, I can understand the plight of the small restaurateurs in America struggling to understand how they would go against the norm of low pay and poor benefits in this industry and still succeed. However, the employers profiled in this book show that norms and standards can evolve in ways that help workers, employers, and consumers to thrive collectively. Times are changing, and the industry—and society—certainly can do better.

HOW WE ARE FORKED

Right now, more than eleven million Americans work in restaurants. Unfortunately, the people who prepare, cook, and serve our food are also twice as likely as other Americans to be on food stamps.[1] The restaurant industry—the industry that feeds us!—is also starving its workforce, both economically and as a civil society that values its citizens. However, this book sets out to describe a different path, which some employers are already on, to resolve these challenges.

Workers, consumers, and even employers have been gouged—"forked"—by low standards for employee treatment that have been set by the largest companies in this industry. But in another sense, the industry is also at a fork in the road: much of the industry is following the "low road" to profitability that has been modeled by a majority of large corporate restaurant chains, whereas a small but growing group of employers have shown that taking the "high road" to profitability results in better payoffs in the long run. In fact, a 2014 study conducted by Cornell University researchers in partnership with ROC shows that employers can cut costly employee turnover almost *in half* by providing higher wages and better working conditions, a tremendous gift to an industry that suffers from one of the highest employee turnover rates of any sector.[2] This book will profile people and companies taking both paths, and show how we can get where we need to go by taking the "high road" at the fork in the road.

This book is a guide for anyone who eats out and anyone who wants to eat out better and more ethically. It is a tool to help us understand how restaurants fare on issues of worker wages, benefits, and promotions. Most importantly, this book (along with ROC's smart phone application—more on this later) gives consumers the tools they need to communicate their values every time they eat out. This book includes both ratings of well-known restaurant companies and more in-depth profiles of companies that rate well and others that do not.

This book is not intended to condemn any companies, organizations, or individuals; on the contrary, the book is meant to show both the challenges at hand and that change is possible anywhere and everywhere, and that change is completely within our power as consumers to effect within our lifetimes.

WHY THIS BOOK?

In 2013, I wrote a book called *Behind the Kitchen Door*, about working conditions in the restaurant industry, then proceeded to take my

4

seven-month-old daughter with me on an insane book tour across the country. We stopped in big and small cities, and I spoke in churches, libraries, bookstores, restaurants, and anyplace that would have us. Sometimes I'd take my daughter with me up to the podium, and other times she'd be crawling around in the back of the audience while I pounded the podium with my fist and described the poverty-level wages and abysmal working conditions faced by the millions of restaurant workers in this country. I would talk about the work of ROC, the national movement that I co-founded and co-direct, and our work over the last twelve years to bring workers, responsible employers, and consumers together to change the industry.

In too many instances, women would approach me at the end of the book talk and share horrific stories of sexual harassment and assault while working as servers in restaurants. These stories dramatically changed the course of ROC's work, as I'll describe later.

Either way, everywhere I spoke, anytime I spoke, people would always ask, "So what can we do?" "Where can we eat?" And someone, almost every single time, would come up with the idea that everyone felt they had discovered for the first time—the idea of a diners' guide, something tangible to tell eaters which restaurants fare well on issues of wages and working conditions for restaurant workers. And I would always say, "Yes, we have an app for that."

The first *ROC Diners' Guide to Ethical Eating* was created for New York City in 2007, and it was a simple booklet to highlight restaurant owners who were providing livable wages and working conditions to their employees. We grew into a national organization that same year, and in 2012, published our first national version of the guide online and as a smartphone app. The guide and app rated the 100 most popular restaurant chains and also provided awards to approximately 75 of our responsible restaurant employer partners.[3]

We never created the guide to tell people where to eat and where not to eat. If every ethical eater in America only frequented the 100 or so restaurants around the country that have been given awards for responsible employment in our app, we would eat in restaurants much less. Instead, we sought to provide a tool for consumers to speak up *wherever* and *whenever* they ate out—to say to managers and owners, "I loved the food, loved the service, and I'd love to keep coming back here. I just wanted to let you know that how a restaurant fares in this app on worker wages, benefits, and promotions practices are important to me as a consumer."

This book represents the next step in that process. The book includes the same ratings of employers' wages, benefits, and promotions practices, but it also includes profiles of restaurants that rate highly and others that rate poorly in specific food and labor categories. It especially tells the stories of outstanding restaurant employers—we call them "high-road" employers because they take the high road to profitability—who are growing and profitable *because* they pay and treat their workers well, not *in spite* of their above-average wages and working conditions. In particular, we focus on how these employers have managed to excel in the categories listed in this book.

We also profile employers who currently take the "low road" to profitability, but all of them have great potential to move over to the high road with some encouragement and pressure from all of us. In creating the *Diners' Guide,* we sought to find a way to create simple, straightforward categories with which to rate restaurants, and realized that we needed to prioritize the key issues that restaurant workers have told us were their most important challenges during the last decade.

WHAT ARE THE KEY ISSUES THIS BOOK RATES?

This book is not an exhaustive examination of all the merits or demerits of various restaurant companies' employment practices.

Instead, it is a tool for consumers to begin to think about what to look for in a restaurant with regard to how it treats its workers. The key issues that workers have prioritized—and thus the ones we discuss in this book—are the same key policies that the Cornell researchers found are key to reducing employee turnover and thus increasing retention, productivity, and customer satisfaction: wages, benefits, and internal mobility, regardless of workers' race or gender.

1. Wages

With almost eleven million workers, the restaurant industry is currently the second-largest and one of the fastest-growing employer sectors in the United States.[4] Nearly one in twelve working Americans works in the restaurant industry right now.[5] The restaurant industry is one of the only sectors to grow amid the economic crisis of the last decade.[6] We have continued to eat out as a nation in ever-increasing numbers, even when we are unemployed.

Unfortunately, while it is one of the largest and fastest-growing segments of the United States economy, it is also the absolute lowest-paying employer in the United States. Every year the U.S. Department of Labor releases a list of all occupations in the United States, including their hourly wages, and every year the restaurant industry wins the prize for having the lowest-paying occupations in the United States. Every year at least six to seven of the ten lowest-paying occupations are restaurant occupations, with only one or two of those occupations being fast-food jobs. Currently, restaurant workers occupy seven of the ten lowest-paid occupations reported by the Bureau of Labor Statistics; at least four of these are in full-service restaurants.[7]

So how is it that one of the largest and fastest-growing sectors of the U.S. economy—clearly a successful sector—is proliferating the nation's lowest-paying jobs? Our analysis is that much of this persisting, extraordinary imbalance can be traced to the power of a trade lobbying group called the National Restaurant Association, which we at ROC call the Other NRA. The Other NRA, led by the nation's Fortune 500 restaurant chains, has been named among Congress's most powerful lobbying groups by *Fortune* Magazine.[8,9] The NRA has lobbied extensively to keep the minimum wage as low as possible; not surprisingly, the restaurant industry is the largest employer of minimum-wage workers in the United States.[10] As a result, the median hourly wage for all restaurant workers in the United States is a paltry $9.20.[11]

Many people assume that low wages in the restaurant industry are concentrated in the fast-food segment of the industry. Unfortunately, this is not the case. Workers in all segments of the industry, in all positions and of all racial and gender backgrounds work and live in poverty in the restaurant industry. Wages for kitchen workers are abysmal, and, unbeknownst to many, income for workers serving customers on the dining floor—workers who earn tips—is no better.

In Chapter 2 of this book, I describe a brief history of tipping and the minimum wage for tipped workers over the last 150 years, and how the current system of allowing the restaurant industry to exempt itself from paying its own workers because they earn tips is a legacy of slavery. Over the last century, the restaurant industry has continuously lobbied for tipping to be entrenched in American restaurant culture and for resultant exemptions from minimum wage laws for restaurant employers.[12] This history climaxed in 1996, when the CEO of the NRA was Herman Cain, a former business analyst for Pillsbury who made his name working for brands such as Burger King and Godfather's Pizza. (Cain would later pursue the 2012 Republican presidential nomination and a 2004 Georgia senatorial nomination, losing in the primaries for both.) In his time at the NRA Cain struck a deal with Congress: the NRA would not oppose a modest increase in the overall minimum wage as long as the minimum wage for tipped workers would in turn stay frozen *forever*. The argument of the NRA was that since these workers earned tips, they should never actually receive a wage increase. The federal minimum wage for tipped workers has thus remained frozen at $2.13 an hour for almost 25 years. The Other NRA thus succeeded in convincing Congress and the American people that it should be the only industry on earth to win an extraordinary exemption for itself, saying that they should not have to pay their own workers' wages but, instead, customers should.[13]

Similar deals have been struck countless times over the last decade in at least forty-four states across the country. Seven states—California, Oregon, Washington, Montana, Alaska, Nevada, and Minnesota—have had the same wages for tipped and nontipped workers for decades.[14] Although the NRA argues that paying tipped and nontipped workers the same minimum wage would put them out of business, eliminate server positions, or reduce customer tipping, none of these predictions has been borne out in the seven states with no mandated lower wage for tipped workers.[15] These seven states actually have faster restaurant-industry job-growth rates, higher job-growth rates (specifically in server occupations), and higher restaurant sales per capita than the forty-three states with lower wages for tipped workers.[16] Tipping averages are the same in these states, and, in fact, Alaska has the highest tipping average of any state in the United States—and is a state with the same wage for tipped and nontipped workers.[17]

So, then, how and why has the Other NRA gotten away with this extraordinary exemption? They've gotten away with it by painting the picture of a young man who works at a fine dining restaurant, earning $18 an hour in tips and living the high life. In reality, two-thirds of tipped workers in America are women, and they largely work at casual restaurants like the Olive Garden, Applebee's, IHOP, and Denny's. Their median wage, including tips, is $8.77 per hour in states with a tipped minimum wage. These women suffer three times the poverty rate of the rest of the United States workforce and use food stamps at double the rate.[18]

As a result of the same deal having been struck between the NRA and state legislators in states across the country, wages for tipped workers in America range between $2.13 and about $5 in forty-one states nationwide.[19] When you are a tipped worker who receives between $2.13 and $5 an hour, you don't actually receive a wage; your wage is so small it goes entirely to taxes, and you get a paystub with $0 that says, "THIS IS NOT A PAYCHECK." As a result, the vast majority of tipped workers in America live completely off their tips, which creates extraordinary economic instability. These workers never know how much they are going to earn from week to week, day to day, or month to month. Although their bills and rent do not fluctuate, their income does.

During my 2013 book tour, women approached me at the end of book talks and shared stories that illustrated how our nation's system of requiring certain workers to live off tips is not simply a matter of economic instability; it's a matter of human indecency. Women related stories of having to objectify themselves to earn enough tips to survive—and since the customer was paying their wages, rather than their employer, the customer was always right. This meant that these women had to tolerate whatever a customer might do to them—however they might touch, treat, or talk to them—because, again, the customer was always right.

This dynamic was eloquently summarized by a restaurant server member of ROC, Amber, who spoke at a Senate press conference in Washington, DC, in 2013. She testified, "Senators, imagine if your income depended on the happiness of the people you serve.

Because my income depends on the happiness of the people I serve, I have to put up with a guy groping my butt every day to feed my four-year-old son at night."

Forcing women to live off tips also means that these women have to objectify themselves to get their tips. I've heard countless stories of women being told by their supervisors to "go home and dress more sexy, show more cleavage!" in order to sell more food and make more money in tips. This practice exposes women to sexual harassment not only from customers but also from co-workers and managers. In fact, the restaurant industry is the single largest source of sexual-harassment complaints to the EEOC of any industry in the United States. Seven percent of American women work in restaurants, but 37 percent of all sexual harassment complaints to the EEOC come from the restaurant industry.[20]

One woman, speaking from the audience at a talk I was giving, related a horrific story of having worked as a server as a young woman. Her manager had taken her into a walk-in freezer, held her at knifepoint, and raped her brutally. She felt she had no choice but to comply, and was forced to finish out her shift afterward.

One of the most personally saddening parts of the stories women were sharing with me was that many had moved on to other professions, but their experiences in the restaurant industry impacted their careers. Multiple women repeated more or less the same story: *I'm a corporate lawyer/executive/professional. I've been sexually harassed recently on the job, but never did anything about it because it was never as bad as it was when I was a young woman working in restaurants.* These stories led us to understand that besides the six million women who must put up with this system daily as restaurant workers, there are millions more women who work in the restaurant industry as their first job in high school, college, or graduate school. In fact, restaurants pride themselves on offering first jobs for most young people. For young women, however, most of them working as tipped workers, having their first jobs in the restaurant industry means that they are introduced into the world of work in a situation in which they are encouraged to sell themselves and their bodies to earn their income. It is the industry through which they learn what is tolerable and acceptable in the workplace—an industry in which they must tolerate the most extremely inappropriate behavior from customers, co-workers, and managers—in order to be able to feed their families.

For all these reasons, over the last few years, ROC has led a campaign to eliminate the lower wage for tipped workers, called One Fair Wage. To be clear, our campaign is to eliminate the lower wage for tipped workers, not tipping altogether; unless and until employers can provide a professional, livable income to their workers, tips are absolutely necessary on top of a full base wage to get workers closer to a wage that will allow them to support their families. Some restaurants have chosen to eliminate tipping altogether; we applaud them if they do so in a transparent manner and ultimately pay their workers a full base wage that is equivalent to what they would have earned through tips.

In this book, we give a restaurant a point if it provides nontipped workers with at least $10 as a starting wage, and another point if it provides tipped workers with more than their state's tipped minimum wage. We also especially commend restaurants moving toward One Fair Wage—eliminating the lower wage for tipped workers altogether.

2. Paid Sick Days

Ninety percent of restaurant workers nationwide report not having paid sick days, and two-thirds report cooking, preparing, and serving our food when they are sick—with everything from H1N1 to Hepatitis A.[21] Restaurant workers not having paid sick days means that they are forced to come to work while sick or risk losing their job. Workers report that they are told that they will be fired if they do not come to work, even if they are sick. Even among those workers who are not told they will be fired, without receiving pay when they are sick, the vast majority of workers prefer to work when sick rather than cutting into an already too-paltry income. As mentioned earlier, too many of these workers live completely off tips, which can only be obtained by physically coming to work.

Of course, the issue is also a public health concern. Sick restaurant workers infect co-workers and, of course, customers. The Centers for Disease Control (CDC) reports that 50–90 percent of all norovirus (stomach flu) outbreaks can be traced back to sick restaurant workers.[22]

Recent efforts across a broad coalition of organizations have pushed paid sick days legislation in states and cities across the country, with tremendous success: seventeen cities, including Washington, DC, and the states of Connecticut, Massachusetts, and California have passed paid sick-days laws.[23] Of course, these victories have not been achieved without intense opposition from the Other NRA, which argues that restaurants will be forced to close, shed jobs, or not grow as quickly if they must provide paid sick days. In fact, in 2013 the Other NRA joined forces with Darden, the world's largest full-service restaurant company and owner of the Olive Garden, Capital Grille Steakhouse, and LongHorn Steakhouse, among other brands. Darden helped write the preemption legislation in Florida, and the Other NRA, where Darden plays a leading role, pushed preemption bills around the country prohibiting any localities in those states from passing local paid-sick-days ordinances. Such preemptive legislation was passed in eight of the fourteen states in which it was introduced, undermining citizens' ability to pass local paid-sick-days legislation even if it was democratically approved by a majority or even a unanimity of voters in a particular locality.[24,25] The current count of preemption states is eleven, with eight having been passed in the last two years.[26]

Nonetheless, the fight to expand paid-sick-days legislation to more cities and states—and thus protect the public health—continues. Many restaurant employer partners and others around the country have implemented paid sick days and found the policy to have enormous benefits in terms of worker productivity and retention. Several are profiled in this book. In this book, we denote restaurants that provide even a single sick day with a thermometer icon (🌡).

3. Internal Mobility

Two-thirds of restaurant workers surveyed nationally reported never receiving a promotion to a higher-paying position, and even fewer reported ever being offered training necessary to move up the ladder to higher-level positions.[27] Although there is a myth of mobility in the industry—the idea that a dishwasher could one day open her own restaurant—the reality is that the vast majority of workers see very little advancement in their careers.

Such lack of advancement has serious racial implications, because the restaurant industry is highly racially segregated. Workers of color are segregated into lower-level segments—fast-food and casual restaurants as opposed to fine dining—and even lower-level positions—kitchen and busser positions rather than server and bartending positions—especially in fine dining restaurants. This results in workers of color earning $4 less per hour than white workers in the U.S. restaurant industry overall.[28]

ROC research shows that although 80 percent of restaurant worker occupations provide poverty-level wages, up to 20 percent of the jobs in the industry *can* provide a livable wage.[29] These are largely server and bartender positions in fine dining restaurants. As mentioned earlier, the majority of servers in America do not work in fine dining restaurants and suffer from three times the poverty rate of the rest of the U.S. workforce. However, servers and bartenders in fine dining restaurants can earn a livable wage; unfortunately, these jobs are held in vast majority by white men.[30] Workers of color face significant barriers in attempting to advance either from lower-level positions in fine dining restaurants or from fast-food or casual restaurants into fine dining.

With so little mobility in the industry, most servers in fine dining restaurants are hired from outside the restaurant, and most are white. In 2014, ROC released a series of matched-pairs audit-testing studies, having sent into fine dining restaurants hundreds of pairs of white and people of color applicants with identical resumes, personalities, and size and height characteristics to see who would be hired as servers. We found that white applicants had twice the chance of a person of color of getting hired as a fine dining server.[31]

In the alternative scenario, several responsible restaurant employers—including several profiled in this book—have chosen to invest in their own workforce by training and promoting workers from within the company to the highest-paying positions in the company. Zingerman's, an Ann Arbor mainstay featured in the "sandwich" chapter of this book, even goes so far as to train and promote workers all the way up to the ownership level.

In this book, we provide a notation (⏏) for any restaurant that has provided a raise or a promotion to a higher-paying position to at least 50 percent of its current staff within the last year. This is a decent measure of mobility, but not a complete measure of racial discrimination and segregation, which requires ongoing study and investigation. Consumers can be a part of observing, documenting,

and changing patterns of racial segregation in the restaurant industry using ROC's smartphone application, as described in greater
detail in this book's conclusion.

LOCAL VERSUS NATIONAL

As mentioned earlier, this book rates restaurants in various food
categories—casual and family-style restaurants, fine dining restaurants, Mexican fast-food restaurants, coffee shops, sandwich restaurants, burgers, and diners. Each chapter of this book focuses on a
different food category, and in each chapter we provide an in-depth
story of a restaurant company that receives a high rating in the category, and another that receives a low rating.

It will not be surprising to some that most of the restaurants
receiving high marks in this book are not national chains, and that
all the restaurants receiving low marks are national chains. (In-N-
Out Burger and Chipotle provide the exception.) Foodies might
be relieved to not see their favorite fine dining restaurant receive a
negative rating in this book; it might be easier for some to condemn
chain restaurants.

However, poverty wages, lack of benefits such as paid sick days,
and a lack of upward mobility are certainly not unique to national
restaurant chains. Unfortunately, these conditions are vastly pervasive throughout the industry, regardless of geography, ownership
structure, or size. We still need to talk to and encourage most of our
favorite local restaurants, because statistics show they are likely following the same low-road standards set by the chains. Nevertheless,
all the restaurants receiving low marks in this book are restaurant
chains for two reasons. First, it would have been impossible to rate
all restaurants in America, and thus we chose to focus on the most
popular restaurants in each category, in addition to those willing

to provide the information requested. Nonchain restaurants willing to provide the information tended to be responsible restaurant owner partners of ROC. Second, and perhaps more important, America's largest chain restaurants lead the National Restaurant Association and lobby to set minimum wage and paid sick days standards in this country. They also set standards with regard to training and mobility. As the restaurant companies that set standards for the industry, they bear the responsibility of additional scrutiny. After all, they could just as well set a higher employment standard for the industry—a standard that most other restaurants in America could follow. It is our hope that they soon will.

Of course, this dichotomy might lead some to question the comparisons. If most of the higher-rated companies are small and local, and most of the lower-rated companies are large and national, couldn't the lower employment standards be related to size and geography? Perhaps, some might say, it is impossible for larger companies to provide higher wages and benefits as they grow. Even if it is not impossible, how can smaller companies provide lessons on doing things differently to larger companies; in other words, can the high employment standards of the smaller companies featured in this book be taken to scale?

I offer a few key responses to these questions. First, In-N-Out Burger and Chipotle rule out the notion that it is impossible to take higher employment standards to scale. Second, smaller companies have fewer advantages than larger companies, not greater. Larger companies have larger profit margins, more liquid cash, and countless economies of scale that would allow them to increase standards more easily than a smaller company with smaller profit margins. If the small companies featured in this book were able to implement higher wage and benefit standards and still survive, even thrive, then, so too, should large national companies be able to follow.

But what about the local versus national question? Several of the high-road employers profiled in this book—Vimala of

Vimala's Curryblossom Café in North Carolina, Zingerman's Community of Businesses, and Andy Shallal, owner of Busboys and Poets and Eatonville—argue that there is an inherent advantage to remaining a local company. All argue that local companies are invested in and integral to local communities and local economies in ways that national companies are not. Fortunately, although the companies that lead the National Restaurant Association in setting industry-wide standards are all national chains, the majority of restaurant companies in America are still smaller local companies that have the potential to be rooted in local communities. This would suggest that our fight must be to ensure that wages and working conditions improve across all different types of restaurants *and* that local restaurants continue to grow and thrive in spite of the growth of national restaurant chains. It would also suggest that local restaurant owners share something with restaurant workers nationwide, in all kinds of restaurants—namely, the need to move the restaurant chains that lead the National Restaurant Association to set different standards for the industry, respecting both workers and their neighbors in local communities.

HOW THIS BOOK WORKS

Each chapter of this book focuses on one type of restaurant and provides both ratings for companies in that restaurant type and profiles of restaurant companies in that restaurant type. In each chapter— and thus for each restaurant type—I provide ratings for the top ten or so most-popular restaurant companies, and also for several high-road employers in that segment. In each, I profile one company that fared well in our rating system, and one that could greatly improve its ratings.

In each chapter, I also highlight a key issue or frame that distinguishes restaurants taking the high road from those taking the low road. The first half of the book highlights each of the issues measured in the guide—wages, promotion practices, and benefits. I start in Chapter 2 with casual and family restaurants, as the epicenter of the battle over America's sordid history of tipping and the lower minimum wage for tipped workers. In Chapter 3, I describe fine dining restaurants, where this battle is exacerbated by severe race and gender segregation and discrimination. In Chapter 4's Mexican fast-food restaurants, I describe internal promotion as a key strategy to overcome some of these challenges, and in Chapter 5's burger restaurant profiles, I distinguish companies that provide paid sick days and livable wages for nontipped workers from those that do not.

The second half of the book describes broader frames that distinguish the high-road perspective from the low-road perspective. Chapter 6 describes two different sandwich restaurant companies that have two very different approaches to growth; Chapter 7 focuses on coffee shops and the space provided for workers to speak up about their conditions and engage in original thinking and debate—the original crux of coffee-shop culture. Finally, Chapter 8 describes American greasy-spoon diners as the epicenters of racial and cultural change—some that prove that any restaurant company can transform itself in ways that benefit workers, consumers, and ultimately the employers themselves.

HOW THE BOOK'S RATING SYSTEM WORKS

Working with students from the University of North Carolina, the University of California, Berkeley, and the University of

Georgia,[32] ROC asked restaurants about their practices with regard to:

1. Wages for tipped workers and nontipped workers.
2. Paid sick leave policy.
3. Actual provision of raises and promotions, a partial measure for internal mobility.

We asked for this information from all of our high-road restaurant partners across the country, and from the top ten highest-revenue-grossing restaurants in the United States in each category of food. Data for assessing the top ten in each restaurant category was taken from the *Nation's Restaurant News'* top 100 lists.[33]

Using this top 100 list at the unit level, students and workers actually visited each restaurant company's individual restaurant locations to inquire about employment conditions. Students focused on individual restaurant locations in the South, where legally required employment standards are the lowest, to understand the lowest standards offered in a particular national or international restaurant company anywhere in the country with regard to wages and paid sick days.[34] Students from the University of California, Berkeley then followed up with phone calls to these same restaurants about the actual provision of raises and promotions.

Restaurants in this book are evaluated in four different areas, and can receive different accreditations based on meeting criteria in each. They receive one point for every criterion met. If a restaurant receives three out of four points, they are awarded one star (★). If the restaurant receives four out of four points, they are awarded two stars (★★).

Different accreditations are indicated with the following symbols:

$10 + Wage for Nontipped Workers: A restaurant receives a point if their lowest starting wage for a nontipped worker is at least $10. Nontipped workers include hosts and hostesses, dishwashers, prep cooks, line cooks, and porters.

(⑤+) Hourly Wage for Tipped Workers Exceeds Minimum: A restaurant receives a point if their lowest starting wage for a tipped worker is higher than the state minimum wage for tipped workers. Tipped workers include servers, runners, bussers, bartenders, barbacks, and expeditors. Although there are seven states that do not have a lower wage for tipped workers, most other states have wages for tipped workers of between $2.13 and $5 per hour. We especially recognize restaurants that are moving toward a higher wage for tipped workers and ultimately, as in the seven states, eliminating the lower wage for tipped workers altogether.

(🕯) Paid Sick Days: A restaurant receives a point if it provides paid sick days to its part-time and full-time employees through a paid-sick-day policy or by policies allowing for paid time off to be used for sick days.

(🔔) Promotion Practices: A restaurant receives a point if at least 50 percent of its current employees have received a raise or a promotion to a higher-paying position in the last year.

HOW YOU CAN USE THIS BOOK

1. Download and share the *ROC Diners' Guide* app.
Download our smartphone app here (rocunited.org/dinersguide) and share it with your friends to help them eat ethically as well. This nifty app uses geolocators to map out *ROC Diners Guide* awarded restaurants around the country. You can also let employers know that you care about how they treat their workers—it's quick and

easy on Twitter and Yelp, and you will help to shift industry standards on things like the racial makeup of people in the highest paid positions.

2. Talk to restaurateurs about your values.
Use this book and the *ROC Diners' Guide* app to start a conversation about your values when you eat out, especially with restaurants that rank poorly in the *Guide* or aren't included yet. I like to say to owners at the end of my meal, "I loved the food. I loved the service. I'd love to keep coming here, but I want you to know that the criteria in this app are important to me. It's important to me to know that your workers are paid a living wage, provided paid sick days, and provided lots of opportunities to move up the ladder, regardless of their race or gender."

3. Eat ethically at a high-road restaurant!
Whenever possible, support the award-winning restaurants in this book. Let them know you support them for their great employment practices. And if you know of a restaurant not listed in the guide that you think might be committed to the high road, let them know about ROC's high-road employer association RAISE (raisewithroc. org), which offers a place for restaurateurs to support one another on that path.

4. Let your elected officials know that we need to eliminate the two-tiered system of a separate, lower wage for tipped workers in favor of One Fair Wage.
You can visit www.rocunited.org to send a letter to your representatives letting them know we also need paid sick days for all workers in America so we won't have to worry about our cooks or servers working when they are sick.

5. Hold low-road employers accountable.
You can help by supporting workers pursuing claims against restaurant employers who have been charged with violating the law.

When you know that workers have complained, as in the case of the Darden Restaurant Group, which owns the Olive Garden and Capital Grille Steakhouse, you can call the company to let them know that you won't support such questionable practices.

6. Join ROC!

We have created an ethical diners' association called Diners United, mobilizing restaurant-goers in support of livable wages and working conditions for the nation's eleven million restaurant workers. Join the growing network of people who care about the food they eat and the people behind it. Visit dinersunited.com, and join us!

NOTES

1. American Community Survey, 2013 (ACS, 2013). Calculations by the Restaurant Opportunities Centers United (ROC United) based on Ruggles et al., *Integrated Public Use Microdata Series: Version 5.0* [Machine-readable database]. (Minneapolis: Minnesota Population Center, 2010).
2. Rosemary Batt, Jae Eun Lee, ILR School, Cornell University, Tashlin Lakhani, Ohio State University, *High Road 2.0: A National Study of Human Resource Practices, Turnover, and Customer Service in the Restaurant Industry.* (New York, NY: ROC United, 2014).
3. "2013 ROC National Diners' Guide to Ethical Eating,", http://thewelcometable.net/dinersguide/ (accessed February 23, 2015).
4. R. Henderson, R. 2012. "Industry Employment and Output Projections to 2020," *Monthly Labor Review* 135 (2012): 65.
5. ACS, 2013.
6. Bureau of Labor Statistics, U.S. Department of Labor, *Current Employment Statistics (CES)*, 2014 [www.bls.gov/ces/]. Employment, hours, and earnings from the CES survey, by industry.
7. Bureau of Labor Statistics, U.S. Department of Labor, *Occupational Employment Statistics (OES)*, 2014 [www.bls.gov/oes/]. National cross-industry estimates sorted by median hourly wage for all standard occupational classifications.
8. Jeffrey H. Birnbaum, The power 25, *Fortune*, 1999.
9. Judy Sarasohn, "Fortune Cookie: You Hit the Top 10," *Washington Post*, November 25, 1999. <http://www.washingtonpost.com/wp-srv/WPcap/1999-11/25/059r-112599-idx.html>

10. "Characteristics of Minimum Wage Workers, 2013," US Bureau of Labor Statistics, Report 1048, March 2014, http://www.bls.gov/cps/minwage2013.pdf.
11. BLS, OES, 2014.
12. Kerry Segrave, *Tipping: An American Social History of Gratuities* (Jefferson, NC: McFarland & Company,1998).
13. Alan Liddle, "Associations Urge Senate to Retain Wage Provisions," *Nation's Restaurant News*, Vol. 30 Issue 25, p. 1, June 24, 1996.
14. ROCUnited.org, "State of Tipped Workers," http://rocunited.org/state_of_tipped_workers/ (accessed February 26, 2015).
15. ROC United, *Recipe for Success: Abolish the Subminimum Wage to Strengthen the Restaurant Industry* (New York, NY: ROC United, 2014).
16. Ibid.
17. Roberto A. Ferdman, "Map: Where Americans Are Generous Tippers," *The Atlantic*, March 21, 2014, http://www.theatlantic.com/business/archive/2014/03/map-where-americans-are-generous-tippers/284567/.
18. ROCUnited.org, "State of Tipped Workers,"
19. Wage and Hour Division (WHD), US Department of Labor, "Minimum Wages for Tipped Employees," USJanuary 1, 2015, http://www.dol.gov/whd/state/tipped.htm.
20. ROC United, Forward Together, *The Glass Floor: Sexual Harassment in the Restaurant Industr.*, (New York, NY: ROC United, 2014).
21. ROC United, *Behind the Kitchen Door: A Multi-Site Study of the Restaurant Industry*, (New York, NY: ROC United, 2011).
22. Centers for Disease Control and Prevention, "Norovirus Is the Leading Cause of Disease Outbreaks from Contaminated Food in the US," http://www.cdc.gov/media/releases/2014/p0603-norovirus.html (accessed February 23, 2015),
23. National Partnership for Women and Families, *"State and Local Action on Paid Sick Days."* Washington, DC, May 2015. http://www.nationalpartnership.org/research-library/campaigns/psd/state-and-local-action-paid-sick-days.pdf
24. Mary Bottari, "The 'Other NRA,' the National Restaurant Association, Pushes Preemption of Paid Sick Days," The Center for Media and Democracy's PR Watch, July 24, 2013, http://www.prwatch.org/news/2013/07/12173/other-nra-national-restaurant-association-pushes-preemption-paid-sick-days.
25. Ashley Lopez, "Florida Senate May Consider House's More Restrictive Anti-Sick Pay Bill," Florida Center for Investigative Reporting, April 25, 2013. http://fcir.org/2013/04/25/florida-senate-may-consider-houses-more-restrictive-anti-sick-pay-bill/?pfstyle=wp.

26. http://www.nationalpartnership.org/issues/work-family/preemption-map.html; http://www.nytimes.com/2015/02/24/us/govern-yourselves-state-lawmakers-tell-cities-but-not-too-much.html.

27. ROC United, *Behind the Kitchen Door: A Multi-Site Study of the Restaurant Industry*, (New York, NY: ROC United, 2011).

28. ROC United, *The Great Service Divide: Occupational Segregation & Inequality in the US Restaurant Industry*, (New York, NY: ROC United, 2014).

29. Ibid.

30. Ibid.

31. Ibid.

32. We thank the students of Professor Aaron Schneider from the University of Denver, and Professor Sarah Stiles from Georgetown University for all their hard work on this project. Specifically, Julie Leebove, Hans Schaler, Erin Orsley, Julia Lopez, and Denise Recinos.

33. "Top 100: Methodology," *Nation's Restaurant News*, http://nrn.com/corporate/top-100-methodology (accessed March 28, 2015).

34. For restaurant chains with multiple locations, we asked about these practices from restaurants within the chain primarily in Alabama, Texas, Louisiana, Mississippi, South Carolina, Tennessee, and Georgia. In all those states, there is no state labor law and only federal labor law applies; thus, wages paid in establishments in those states would be the lowest wage paid by the restaurant chain anywhere in the country.

[2]

CASUAL AND FAMILY-STYLE
RESTAURANTS

Family-style casual restaurants have become ubiquitous in every sector of America. They are the moderately priced, family-friendly outposts that populate the middle ground between fast food and fine dining, and they're where 99 percent of diners take their families to eat when not cooking at home.

Casual and family-style restaurants are also the epicenter of the U.S. restaurant industry's fork in the road. As the largest employers of tipped workers, they are the front lines in the battle over tipping and the lower minimum wage for tipped workers.

Several casual restaurant chains in the United States epitomize the challenges of the tipping system in America. Each of the full-service casual restaurant chains listed in Table 2.1 pays servers a minimum wage as low as $2.13 an hour for tipped workers.

There are some casual restaurants that are bucking the trend (Table 2.2), leading the high road for this sector of American dining.

Table 2.1 LOW-ROAD RESTAURANTS

	$10+ Wage for Non-tipped Workers	Hourly Wage for Tipped Workers Exceeds Minimum	Paid Sick Days	Promotion Practices	Stars
BJ's Restaurant and Brewhouse					
California Pizza Kitchen					
Carrabba's Italian Grill	💵				
Cheddar's					
Cheesecake Factory					
Logan's Roadhouse					
Long Horn Steakhouse	💵				
Olive Garden					
Texas Roadhouse					
TGI Friday's					

Table 2.2 HIGH-ROAD RESTAURANTS

	$10+ Wage for Non-tipped Workers	Hourly Wage for Tipped Workers Exceeds Minimum	Paid Sick Days	Promotion Practices	Stars
1905 Washington, DC	💵		🌡	←	★★
The Original Ben's Chili Bowl Washington, DC		n/a*	🌡	←	★
Busboys & Poets Washington, DC			🌡	←	★
Colors Restaurant Detroit, MI	💵	$+	🌡	←	★★
Dimo's Pizza Chicago, IL			🌡	←	★
Flava at WaZobia Washington, DC				n/a	

(continued)

Table 2.2 CONTINUED

	$10+ Wage for Non-tipped Workers	Hourly Wage for Tipped Workers Exceeds Minimum	Paid Sick Days	Promotion Practices	Stars
Girard *Philadelphia, PA*	💵	n/a*	🌡	n/a	★
Good Restaurant *New York, NY*			🌡	←	★
Inspire BBQ *Washington, DC*	💵	n/a*	🌡	←	★★
Juniper *Wellesley, MA*				n/a	
Kainbigan *Oakland, CA*	💵	💲+		←	★★
Levy Restaurants at Ford Field *Detroit, MI*	💵	n/a*	🌡		★
Lil Dizzy's Café *New Orleans, LA*	💵		🌡	n/a	★

	💵	💲+		🌡	➤	★
Local *Los Angeles, CA*	💵	💲+		🌡	➤	★★
Marietta *Brooklyn, NY*	💵			🌡	➤	★★
Peaches Hothouse *Brooklyn, NY*	💵			🌡	➤	★★
Peaches Restaurant and Bar *Brooklyn, NY*	💵			🌡	➤	★★
So Crepe *Philadelphia, PA*				n/a	n/a	
Snow & Co *Kansas City, MO*	💵			🌡	➤	★★
The Just Crust *Cambridge, MA*	💵	💲+		🌡	n/a	★★

(continued)

Table 2.2 CONTINUED

	$10+ Wage for Non-tipped Workers	Hourly Wage for Tipped Workers Exceeds Minimum	Paid Sick Days	Promotion Practices	Stars
The Quick Fixx Philadelphia, PA	💵			←	★★
The Park's Finest Los Angeles, CA	💵	💲+		n/a	★
The Salty Pig Boston, MA	💵			←	★
The Smoke Joint Brooklyn, NY	💵		🌡	←	★★
Vimala's Curryblossom Café Chapel Hill, NC	💵	n/a*	🌡	←	★★

* No tipped employees.

THE TIPPED MINIMUM
WAGE: A LEGACY OF SLAVERY

According to *Tipping: An American Social History of Gratuities*, by Kerry Segrave, tipping began in the grand Tudor homes of England, where visiting guests were expected to leave gratuities for servants. The custom spread throughout Europe, and expanded from the homes of aristocrats to restaurants and pubs. Wealthy traveling Americans brought the custom to the United States to show they knew the rules, but the custom was seen as despicable, undemocratic, and wholly un-American for decades. An American antitipping movement led by both labor and consumer advocates advocated for an end to tipping; it was seen as giving certain employers the unfair justification that they should be able to pay their workers little or nothing because they were receiving tips. The movement won antitipping legislation in several states, including southern states like South Carolina, Arkansas, Tennessee, and Mississippi. The movement also declared the practice undemocratic to consumers, who should be able to receive quality service regardless of how much they could afford to tip.[1]

Nevertheless, American hospitality and railway companies (the Pullman company in particular) fought to keep the tipping system as it was. In the late 1800s, they argued that they should not have to pay wages to their employees—many of whom were former African-American slaves hired to serve newly industrialized white factory workers in restaurants and traveling Americans on trains—because these workers were earning tips. In other words, the impetus for these industries to be able to hire workers and not pay them a wage at all, arguing that their income could come entirely from customer tips, arose in part from nation's history of subjugation based on race. Segrave quotes 1902 journalist John Speed, who stated on his first trip to the North:

> I had never known any but negro servants. Negroes take tips, of course; one expects that of them—it is a token of their inferiority. But to give money to a white man was embarrassing to me. I felt defiled by his debasement and servility. I do not now comprehend how any native-born American could consent to take a tip. Tips go with servility, and no man who is a voter in this country is in the least justified in being in service."[2]

The Pullman car porters organized an independent union, the Brotherhood of Sleeping Car Porters, and won higher wages before tips.[3] Hospitality workers, however, continued to earn little or no wages from their employers; their income remained entirely dependent on tips.[4] To justify this practice, restaurant employers used much the same argument for more than a century: tipped workers make enormous sums of money in tips, and thus their employers should not have to pay them, practically at all. Throughout that period, the fact that most tipped workers lived in extreme poverty, even with tips, was mostly ignored.[5]

Meanwhile, back in Europe, the antitipping movement picked up and spread quickly. Many Italian hoteliers charged 10–15 percent more in lieu of tipping. "Guests were warned not to tip; employees caught receiving gratuities were fired. At first, the workers were not in favor of the new system, but soon they favored it in both Switzerland and Italy."[6] The practice spread from Italy to Switzerland and France. Traveling Americans threatened to undermine the new system. "You Americans came along and persisted in giving tips as usual,' even though hotel men told the Americans not to give tips."[7] Nevertheless, Italy and Europe continued to move in a no-tipping direction. Italian dictator Mussolini banned tips being accepted from guests at hotels; the practice was seen as servile. During this same period and beyond, America moved in the opposite direction, entrenching tipping and tips into custom and law.

In the United States, the practice of tipping has been institutionalized through a wage system that not only created a justification for the restaurant industry to not have to raise wages for its own workers, but has also very nearly led to the industry arguing that they should not have to pay their workers at all. When Congress passed the first minimum wage law in 1938 as part of the New Deal, the law said that the wage could be obtained through wages or tips; in other words, tipped workers were not guaranteed a base wage from their employers.[8] In 1966 worker advocates were able to win a guaranteed base wage for tipped employees to be paid by their employers, but they were guaranteed only 50% of the overall minimum wage.[9]

Over the next fifty years, Congress ensured that the minimum wage for tipped workers always rose when the minimum wage rose, at a percentage of the overall minimum wage, reaching 60% of the overall minimum wage in 1980.[10] This changed in 1996, however, when the National Restaurant Association reached the height of its power on the issue. Under the leadership of former Godfather's Pizza head Herman Cain, the National Restaurant Association essentially struck a deal with Congress, arguing that they would not oppose a very modest minimum wage increase for other workers as long tipped workers' wages remain frozen forevermore, no longer increasing with the overall minimum wage.[11] Thus, the federal minimum wage for tipped workers was frozen at $2.13 an hour, and has not increased for more than two decades to the current day.[12] Thus, the federal minimum wage for tipped workers has gone from $0, in the first minimum wage law passed in 1938, to $2.13, over a period of almost 80 years.

This same deal struck by the National Restaurant Association has been repeated dozens of times in the United States over the last several decades—deals in which even workers' advocates acceded to a compromise with legislators and the National Restaurant Association. The compromise specified that the minimum wage would increase for all workers as long as tipped workers were left out of the increase. Although seven states maintain the same wage for tipped and nontipped workers, 43 states thereby allow restaurants to pay their workers less than the minimum wage, as little as $2.13, depending on the state.[13] The National Restaurant Association has thus succeeded in convincing many that working people should have to pay other working people's wages through tips.[14-15]

The seven states that have required restaurant employers to pay their workers the full minimum wage regardless of whether they earn tips are California, Oregon, Washington, Nevada, Montana, Alaska, and Minnesota. ROC's research shows that these seven states fare better than the other forty-three on almost every measure the restaurant industry cares about: overall restaurant sales per capita, job growth in the restaurant industry, job growth among tipped workers, and even rates of tipping higher in these seven states.[16,17] This is important, because the Other NRA has spent countless resources trying to convince workers in most states that, if they received the full minimum wage from their own employer, customers would stop tipping them. However, data shows that customers do not tip any less in states that require restaurants to pay the full minimum wage; in some cases they actually tip better. Alaska actually has the highest tipping rates of any state in the United States, and it has required employers to pay the same wage to tipped and nontipped workers for decades.[18] So why couldn't every state do the same?

A large part of the NRA's success in convincing legislators that their members should be exempt is due to their argument that tipped workers receive a more than sufficient income through their tips.[19] The typical portrait is a white man working in a fine dining restaurant, earning $16–$22 an hour in tips. In fact, 66 percent of the almost six million tipped workers in America are women; a large majority work at casual restaurants like the Olive Garden, Applebee's, and IHOP. Tipped workers' median wage including tips is $9.08 an hour; [20] these women suffer three times the poverty rate of the rest of the U.S. workforce and use food stamps at double the rate of the rest of the U.S. workforce.[21]

Thus, the consuming public subsidizes full-service restaurants in two ways: by paying their workers' wages through tips, and by paying for their employees' survival through public assistance. ROC's research shows that half of all full-service restaurant workers use public assistance, for a total of $9.5 billion annually, and that the average Olive Garden, for example, costs the taxpayer nearly $200,000 annually in public assistance for workers.[22]

THE TIPPED MINIMUM WAGE AND SEXUAL HARASSMENT

Earning the subminimum wage for tipped workers most often means living completely off tips. Workers who earn a wage that is as little as $2.13 an hour find that their wages go entirely to taxes, and they are thus completely dependent on tips for income. This dependency creates an untenable economic situation: workers' income fluctuates by year, season, week, shift, and hour. It also fluctuates with the varied whims of customers.

Most pernicious of all, a research study conducted by ROC and Forward Together has shown that workers' dependence on tips for income—especially for women—can exacerbate the already high levels of sexual harassment that occur in the restaurant industry. [23]

Dependent on tips, workers must tolerate whatever a customer might do—treatment, touching, and other behavior—to receive their income from that customer rather than from their employer. Eighty percent of the almost seven hundred restaurant workers surveyed reported experiencing sexual harassment in their restaurant workplace, and 50 percent experienced sexual behaviors that were scary or unwanted. Worst of all, women in states that paid the tipped-worker minimum (often $2.13 an hour) experienced *twice* the rate of sexual harassment from customers as they did in states that paid the same wage to tipped and nontipped workers. Furthermore, women in the states that paid the tipped minimum reported that they were *three times more likely* to be told by their employers to objectify themselves—dressing "sexier," showing more cleavage or wearing tighter clothing—to increase income in tips, because workers in states in which employers pay the full minimum base wage to everyone. In sum: our research showed that when workers were not reliant on customers for a base wage, they were less likely to be sexually harassed.[24]

In Italy and most of Europe, restaurant workers are considered professionals. There are schools of service throughout Europe that train individuals in the art and skill of hospitality.[25] As professionals, many restaurant workers in Europe see it as an affront to offer tips; the practice is demeaning, in the same way that offering a tip to a doctor, professor, or other valued professional would be demeaning in the United States. These professionals demand a livable income from their employer, rather than have to pander to customers, regardless of their behavior.

The de-valuing and de-humanizing of tipped workers in America does not only impact six million workers who currently work for tips. As the first job for most young women in America, the restaurant industry trains young women in what is acceptable and tolerable in the workplace. Most tipped workers are not youth;

they are working adults, many with children. But for the many millions who start in this industry as young people, the experience has lasting impact. As a result, women who move on from this industry into other professions reported that they never did anything about being sexually harassed on the job, because it was never as bad as it had been when they were young and working in restaurants.

For all of these reasons, ROC has led a recent campaign called One Fair Wage to eliminate the lower wage for tipped workers. Through our campaign, numerous states have introduced legislation to eliminate the lower wage for tipped workers. In part as a result of this campaign, there are many restaurants moving in a different direction—moving to eliminate the lower wage for tipped workers altogether, and pay their own workers a full base wage.

One such restaurant is Umi Sushi. General Manager Taki Tanaka came to the United States from Japan at the age of 14, when his father's company transferred him to Chicago. He attended high school and college in the Midwest. "It was interesting; there was no Japanese food anywhere, and that hurt." A sports fan, Tanaka ended up getting a job with Turner Broadcasting Systems in Atlanta as a researcher helping to produce coverage of the 1988 Winter Olympic Games in Japan. Sports television production took him to Connecticut. When the shows he was working on went bust, Tanaka turned to restaurants.

As a server in a Japanese restaurant, Tanaka earned no wage at all and lived off tips. "It was interesting for me, coming from a corporate situation. It was completely different. The payscale was shocking. Basically I thought, 'this is just the way this industry is.'" The owners of the restaurant were immigrants who did not know how to use the computer systems or maintain proper records; Tanaka offered to help them as a manager. He had just begun to set up proper record-keeping systems for the restaurant when a couple who were regulars in the restaurant asked if he would help them open their new sushi restaurants. Since they were offering to sponsor him for a green card, Tanaka could not refuse.

After one failed restaurant, Tanaka and his new partners found success in Umi Sushi, a sushi restaurant they set up near Hartford. Tanaka worked closely with the owners' son to set up all the new rules of the restaurant. "He and I always questioned standard industry practices." Tanaka started the restaurant paying servers $5.15, the minimum wage for tipped workers in Connecticut, but quickly realized that he did not like the system, and decided a few years ago to instead pay servers the full Connecticut minimum wage of $9.15.

"I was really looking at it from a manager's perspective. I thought, 'I want my servers to execute a certain plan that I make.' With tipping, the servers are not really working for me; they're working for an individual customer who will be paying not for service. They're paying for a cute girl or guy. The server may somehow present the table with a freebie, which is a cost to restaurant, to get a higher tip. Bartenders do that all the time. We all try to monitor that as restaurateurs. It's a waste of time. I'd rather have a good system in place, with everybody working as a team, everyone trusting each other, working as a unit, rather than one individual doing whatever he or she wants to do. To do that, I need to be able to reward good work, I need to be able to define what good work is. Not the customers. Customers can say things to me, suggest things, but I need to be able to reward good work, not the customer. Coming from a corporate situation, this part of the restaurant industry doesn't make sense."

THE LOW ROAD: OLIVE GARDEN

With their claim, "When you're here, you're family," Olive Garden has become synonymous with America's proliferation of family-style restaurants. Olive Garden is the largest retail brand of Darden Restaurants, the world's largest full-service restaurant conglomerate, and the world's largest employer of tipped employees. Beyond size, however, Olive Garden has made a name for itself by using the casual or family-style restaurant concept to bring Tuscan-style Italian cuisine to the mainstream. However, there is at least one way in which the Olive Garden and many chain Italian restaurants serving Italian food in America are antithetical to restaurant culture in Italy—through the practice of tipping.[26]

Unlike the other large chain restaurant corporations profiled in this book, there is no hometown origin story, no hometown founder who started poor and made it big, for Olive Garden. The company began in 1982 as a brand-expansion experiment by the food manufacturing and food-service conglomerate General Mills, Inc., and quickly grew into the largest chain of Italian-themed full-service restaurants in the United States. In 1995 General Mills spun off its restaurant holdings into a separate corporation, Darden Restaurants.[27] Darden's growth was based, at least in part, on "using assembly-line methods like those employed at the company's fast-food counterpart, McDonald's."[28]

Darden Restaurants is today the largest full-service directly owned restaurant company in the world. The company originally consisted of Red Lobster, then Olive Garden, then later grew to include Capital Grill Steakhouse, LongHorn Steakhouse, and other popular American brands. (In 2014, in response to a hedge-fund takeover effort, the company sold off Red Lobster.) Olive Garden accounts for $3.6 billion in annual sales and brings in approximately 58 percent of Darden Restaurants' total revenue since the Red Lobster sale. Olive Garden is also Darden's largest chain in terms of employees and locations: of the company's 150,000 workers, 96,000 (64 percent) work at one of Olive Garden's 831 locations in the United States.[29] Olive Garden is also Darden's most value-oriented chain, with an average check of $16.75 per person (versus $72 per person at Capital Grille).[30]

Troubled Times

Olive Garden's sales have begun to decline. The restaurant chain's sales of $3.64 billion in fiscal year 2014 were 1.1 percent below those of fiscal year 2013. The decrease in sales is also reflected in guest counts, which decreased 4.2 percent over the same period.[31] According to *The Business Insider*, Olive Garden is facing fierce competition from fast-casual restaurants like Panera and Chipotle, brands that offer guests lower price points, design that "feels fresher," and food that "is just better."[32] The company has suffered various setbacks in their recent attempts to bring customers back; in 2011, Olive Garden faced criticism and even mockery for offering dishes with inauthentic names such as "pastachetti" and "soffateli." The restaurant chain attributed its declining sales to these unfamiliar menu items.[33] As a result of all these issues, and with an impending hedge- fund takeover, in 2014, Darden announced it would "sell Red Lobster and focus on fixing Olive Garden."[34]

In spring 2014, Darden announced a "brand renaissance" to address the sales crisis at Olive Garden. It involved a new logo for the chain, a countrywide store remodel, and a new menu. Under the outgoing management's plan, seventy-five locations were to receive the new look in 2015, and all Olive Garden locations were to be renovated at a cost of up to $600,000 a piece.[35]

As part of its campaign to gain control of Darden, a hedge-fund called Starboard Value authored a strong critique of Olive Garden's brand-renaissance plan. Starboard pointed toward poor reception of the new Olive Garden logo and the fact that a similar plan had failed to turn around Red Lobster.[36] Starboard also performed an analysis of Olive Garden's ratings on Yelp to demonstrate that the company rates below its peer group, and actually rates the lowest in Middle American states, which constitute the brand's core customer base.[37]

In September 2014, Starboard presented its three-hundred-page report about Darden Restaurants to Darden shareholders, focusing much of its critique around mismanagement at Olive Garden. The report was part of its attempt to convince shareholders to let them take over control of the company. Starboard argued that the Olive Garden suffers from an overly complex menu exemplified by idiosyncratic items like hummus, tapas, and burgers, which confuse the Italian focus of brand. Starboard has also criticized the planned Olive Garden remodel program, arguing that the $175 million planned for the project would destroy shareholder value, and that improving operations and guest experience would be a better emphasis than spending capital on remodels.[38]

Much of Starboard's proposal to cut costs and turn the Olive Garden around focused on cutting labor costs. The group promised it would increase part-time work, buy more prepared food (thus eliminating at least one prep cook per Olive Garden restaurant), and shift more work to tipped employees earning the tipped minimum wage. In proposing this, Starboard inadvertently magnified one of the major negative side effects of a two-tiered wage system, in which tipped workers can be paid as little as $2.13 an hour: employers have a perverse incentive to try to have more tipped employees, and fewer nontipped, and to push as much work onto tipped workers as possible—even when that involves skirting the limits of the applicable legal definitions.

Through these and other cost-saving measures, Starboard argued that the company could realize $36 million annually in labor-cost savings.[39] What these cost-savings projections do not take into account are the enormous costs to thousands of workers: the proposal could mean the loss of between 831 and 1253 positions at

Olive Garden's 831 restaurants, along with immeasurable income lost as greater onus is transferred to the tipping customers.[40]

Takeover

Just before the October 2014 shareholder showdown, Darden's sitting board made a final attempt to win shareholder favor and prevent Starboard from taking over. The company fired three of its top executives, but provided them millions of dollars in severance pay. The Institute for Policy Studies (IPS) produced a shocking report on the company's golden parachutes.

> Darden Restaurants will pay outgoing CEO Clarence Otis a weekly salary of more than $23,000 for the next two years as part of a $2.4 million severance. With multi-million-dollar gains on his stock options and the accrued balance of his company retirement account, Otis' total "golden parachute" amount comes to about $36 million. Two other top executives are walking away with $21 million and $11 million "golden parachutes" of their own, including a combined $2.4 million in severance payments directly from Darden.[41]

When compared to the thousands of the company's employees living daily off an unpredictable income from tips, the severance seems unimaginable. Darden has admitted that it pays at least 20 percent of its U.S. workforce no more than the federal tipped minimum of $2.13 per hour[42,43], and none of these workers could count on retirement funds, even if they worked for the company for a lifetime— let alone severance pay if they were let go for alleged misconduct. The severance pay was especially shocking given the company's vitriolic lobbying efforts to keep wages for workers as low as $2.13. As the IPS study noted, "Since 2008, Darden has spent an average of $1.3 million each year to defeat legislation promoting higher wages and better working conditions."[44]

In the end, despite all the efforts made by Darden board to make changes that would stave off complete hedge-fund takeover, the shareholders voted the entire board out of office and in favor of Starboard management. As challenging as conditions have been for workers under Darden's previous management, the future seems even more uncertain under the management of a hedge-fund that has proposed focusing on severely cutting labor costs as a key solution to the company's financial woes.

Working at Olive Garden While Sick

The Centers for Disease Control estimates that infected restaurant workers are implicated in 70 percent of all norovirus outbreaks—better known as the winter stomach flu—from contaminated food with a known etiology.[45] The Olive Garden does not provide earned sick leave to its employees, which means that workers do not have the right to take a day off when sick and receive pay. This policy is relevant when considering the several illness outbreaks in multiple Olive Garden locations:

In 2006, more than three hundred people complained of norovirus symptoms, known as the winter stomach flu, after eating at an Olive Garden in Indianapolis. The affected diners complained about nausea, vomiting, diarrhea, and fever.[46] Three Olive Garden workers and one customer tested positive for norovirus, according to health officials.[47] Darden settled a class action lawsuit linked to the outbreak for $387,000.[48,50]

Perhaps the most egregious illness outbreak, apparently from sick Olive Garden workers, occurred in 2011, the same year that

Michelle Obama recognized Olive Garden[51] for serving healthy food for children. In 2011, a server in a Fayetteville, North Carolina, Olive Garden worked while ill with Hepatitis A, potentially exposing thousands of customers. With Darden's policy of not providing earned sick leave, and with the minimum wage for servers in North Carolina being $2.13, the server likely could not afford to take a day off despite her illness. The Cumberland County Health Department called in thousands of area diners to be tested for Hepatitis A.[49] After several thousand of these consumers filed a class action lawsuit, Darden settled the case by creating a $375,000 fund to compensate the consumers.[50]

Workers' Rights Violations at Olive Garden

The Olive Garden and its parent company, Darden Restaurants, have been at the center of dozens of lawsuits by employees claiming that their rights were violated. Since 2005, Darden has paid over $14 million to settle lawsuits from servers around wage and hour violations at Olive Garden and Red Lobster.[51]

In 2005, Darden Restaurants agreed to pay $9.5 million to more than twenty thousand current and former servers at California Red Lobster and Olive Garden restaurants in order to settle a lawsuit that alleged violations of state labor regulations when management prevented workers from taking required breaks and required them to purchase and maintain their uniforms.[52] In 2008, Darden Restaurants, Inc. agreed to pay $4 million to settle "two class action lawsuits involving California employees of Red Lobster and Olive Garden restaurants. The suits accused the company of requiring servers and bartenders to make up for cash shortages at the end of their shifts."[53] In 2008, Darden paid $700,000 to settle a wage-dispute lawsuit filed by a former Olive Garden Server in California. The server alleged that "Olive Garden had failed to properly make minimum shift payment and pay minimum wage."[54] In 2011, the U.S. Labor Department found that Olive Garden workers in Mesquite, Texas were not being paid for all their hours. The Department of Labor's investigation concluded that workers were not allowed to clock in at the start of their scheduled work shifts, but rather when customers were seated. Darden agreed to pay $25,000 in back wages to 140 current and former servers. The company was also fined $30,800 in civil money penalties.[55] In 2012, several class action suits were filed against Darden restaurants for underpaying thousands of servers at many restaurants, including Olive Garden.[56]

In addition to these settlements, Olive Garden has tried to implement a number of employment policies that have met with significant worker and public protest. In 2011, Olive Garden implemented a mandatory tip-sharing program, which enabled them to cut more bussers and bartenders hourly wages to $2.13 an hour.[57] This was one of the primary grievances that fueled the growth of ROC's Dignity at Darden campaign, a national coalition of Darden workers, largely from Olive Garden, demanding change in the company. In 2012, Olive Garden experimented with avoiding federal healthcare-reform-related costs by increasing the share of part-time employees in their workforce, but it withdrew the plan under public backlash.[58]

Based on ROC's research linking the tipped minimum wage to sexual harassment, it would follow that Darden and Olive Garden—the largest employer of tipped workers in the United States—would hypothetically be the target of numerous sexual-harassment complaints. As a practical matter, this is difficult to track. The company has instituted a mandatory arbitration policy that requires all employees to sign an agreement that they will utilize a mandatory internal dispute resolution procedure rather than take their claims to court. This has made it more difficult for victims of harassment to bring their claims forward in court—and to track these occurrences and their frequency.

Olive Garden's internal reporting policy has proven to be effective in getting claims dismissed. For example, in 2000, a former Olive Garden employee brought suit against Darden Restaurants alleging that the company "unlawfully subjected her to sexual harassment and a hostile work environment at her place of employment."[59] The case was dismissed because the employee failed to use the company's internal dispute resolution procedure. In another 2012 Missouri-based sexual harassment suit, Darden used the same process argument and the Court agreed.[60]

In some cases, however, the allegations have been so strong that workers and their allies have found other ways to bring the sexual harassment to light. In 2011, the National Action Network called on major investors to disinvest from Darden Restaurants after it was alleged that a "Cleveland-area Olive Garden sexually harassed women, discriminated against new moms, hired [undocumented workers] and didn't adequately discipline a manager who had sex with employees."[61] Employees also alleged that their hours were cut after returning from maternity leave, and that "managers kept a chart rating women by their physical attributes." Darden's email response denied the allegations and claimed that "Darden has a strong, values-based culture built on treating everyone with dignity and respect . . . our company is committed to diversity and our track record speaks for itself."[62]

Olive Garden Case Study: April

April (not her real name) grew up in a single-parent household in a small town in southwest Michigan. During April's childhood, her mother worked in a variety of different industries, including restaurants. April's primary caregivers were her grandmother and aunt, who filled in while her mother was working. "It was a constant struggle. All the time it was hard to put food on the table. Being in that position now, I understand how difficult it can be to be a young woman working as a server and feeding a family."

April remembers wanting to be a server like her mother. "When I was really little, I had a cash register. I would pretend I was a waitress, and go and take everybody's orders. I'd go and get my plastic food. I thought it was the coolest thing in the world, because that's what my mom did."

April says she now understands how little her mother made on tips, and how unsustainable it was.

In 1998, April's mother earned as a server the exact same wage April earns today, almost 20 years later: $2.13 an hour. "The way that inflation is, it might have been easier then to make ends meet on that wage. Now with $2 an hour, maybe I could buy a gumball."

Starting in Restaurants
When April was 16 and old enough to work, she found a job as a hostess at Pizza Hut. "The management was terrible. When I first started, the manager would say, 'OK, I'm going to go tanning and be back in a half of hour,' and leave me and the cook to open the store. I moved from hostess to server, and even turned into the delivery driver, because I just wasn't making enough money."

These financial pressures became more difficult when April became pregnant at 17. After continuing to work at Pizza Hut for a year following the birth of her son, she ended up taking a position at an Olive Garden location near her home. The financial implications of working as a server were immediately clear.

"I had to go back to living with my mom. I couldn't keep paying my bills as a server at the Olive Garden. People don't understand what it's like to be a server. My paycheck is not guaranteed. I live off tips. If I have a table of 20, and they give me a $10 tip, that means I'd have spent three hours waiting on a table hand and foot for $10.

One of the biggest problems for April at Olive Garden was a coworker named Brandon (not his real name). "He wasn't a manager; he was a 'service professional.' He'd say, 'I'm a veteran in this business. I'm a great server.' He had a huge head, and I guess he felt like he wouldn't get in trouble for touching these girls. I guess he was right. He would go around and act like our boss, do whatever he wanted, make lewd statements at these women, grope them. At the Christmas party, he cornered a girl, saying weird things, grabbing her hips. He told another woman, 'I couldn't even tell you what I'm going to do to you.' He got one bartender cornered, and felt her up."

What about Olive Garden's policies for employees to report harassment and other offenses through internal channels? April says these reporting lines are perilous, often stifled by store management through threats of termination if the claims were not substantiated. April heard about what happened from coworkers.

"The women would come out of the office in tears. Pretty soon they'd say, 'I'm done with this. I don't want to give any statement anymore.' Some workers even complained to the regional manager. It was understood that the company had a 'zero tolerance' of sexual harassment policy; it was all over the employee manual and you had to sign a release when you were hired." One of April's male coworkers got in trouble for complaining, but "[Brandon] is still there."

"Those women [who complained] are all gone—they quit or got fired." One of April's male coworkers encouraged them to file a complaint with the EEOC, even anonymously, but they refused. "[Management] scared the hell out of them."

April learned to ignore sexual harassment from customers as a result. "They'll cat call, or say 'She's got a really nice ass.' I've brushed it off. If I was to tell one of my managers, they'd say just brush it off, or just ignore it. It's only when a guest is disturbing other guests, that's when the manager steps up."

April describes how the sexual harassment emanates from a culture in which women are selling themselves to get their income in tips. "Sometimes I've noticed better looking servers get more tips. That's what it's all about. Yes we're serving, and yes, it's about food. But when people go out, they don't want an unattractive server. They want someone who's going to make them feel good about themselves, flirt a little. It's not a gentleman's club, but people still think in the service industry, that we're supposed to meet those personal needs.

"If I don't wear makeup to work, I don't make money."

Serving While Sick

The same disregard for employee well-being extends, April says, to the normalized practice of working and handling food while ill.

"I have tried to call in sick. One time my son was really sick. I called the store, the general manager was there, he answered. I said, 'Hi, my son [is] really sick, I won't be able to make it into the shift. The GM said I needed to find someone to cover me, or work. I couldn't find anyone; it was awful. I was trying to take care of my vomiting child while trying to call people and see if they'd take my shift. In the end, my son's father took him to [the] hospital while I went to work. That was very hard. I ended up being late to work anyway. I went, but I had to wait for my son's dad before I could leave."

Olive Garden's absence of paid sick days has daily, ongoing consequences in April's work there. "I have seen quite a few people working while sick—they have a fever, or they're hacking up a lung, or they have sneezing fits constantly. When someone quits or gets fired, we're not told why. All they do is they'll put up a sign asking if we'd cover shifts because these people no longer wish to work with us. I know one girl had an asthma attack while working there, and that was her last shift. We never saw her again. I don't think they offered her any kind of help, they probably told her to go back on the floor. That's what I think they would do."

April remains a server at Olive Garden, and she's become a leader in ROC to try to help change the industry. "I don't manage [getting by] on tips. I'm trying to save money so that I can get out of my mom's house. She's paying the rent and bills. I provide myself and my son with food, pullups, babywipes, the other basic necessities for living. And that's it. I put gas in my car. And that's all I can do. I cannot afford to live on my own. I have to pay a babysitter. Waiting tables is never going to be enough unless something is done. That's what ROC is all about."

THE HIGH ROAD: VIMALA'S CURRYBLOSSOM CAFE

Like the story of the Olive Garden worker who was forced to work with Hepatitis A, the story of Vimala's Curryblossom Café also takes place in North Carolina—but presents a diametrically opposite picture of working in a North Carolina restaurant. Some reporters have called Vimala's story the story of the "new South;" I call it the story of a new restaurant industry, and a new America.

Vimala Rajendra grew up in Bombay, India, in a home that emphasized gratitude, humility, equality, and respect. These values weren't just platitudes; they were embodied in the way Rajendra's parents lived their lives: "It was not just that my dad respected his boss, or that my mom respected her husband. It went every which way in our family. My father respected, honored, and praised his wife, even when there was a norm against that. He had two daughters before he had a son. He showed so much respect for feminine beauty and brains. He bragged about his daughters' intelligence. He had an uncompromising respect for life, even for the servants who swept our floors. He would ask them if they wanted a cup of tea; they were allowed to sit and drink in our house. It was second nature to us; we would not do it any other way. These values were rooted for my family in our Christian principles; we were Christian. We lived it out."

Also a priority in the Rajendra household: education. Vimala was home schooled, then finished high school at 15 and moved on to earn a bachelor's degree with honors in political science, then taking additional coursework towards a masters degree.

Near the end of her graduate studies, love intervened and brought her to the United States: "I willfully and without the permission of my parents married a man who was ambitious in his scientific career. I left without finishing my masters degree. I came to United States eight months pregnant, and gave birth to [our] first daughter in November after arriving in August."

The transience of her husband's academic career took Rajendra (and the couple's two children) from city to city in the United States and Canada before finally settling in Durham, North Carolina. Once settled, Rajendra returned to school to earn a master's degree in education and, in spite of visa limitations that forbade her from working, took consulting positions with local public television.

As Rajendra became rooted in her North Carolina community, her relationship with her husband became violent. According to Rajendra, "It was too much for him to see me integrated with American society. It drove him crazy. He started beating me, and threatening to beat the girls. Our marriage was becoming a ticking time bomb."

After two years of this alleged abuse and visits from police, Rajendra and her two children left. "First we stayed with a neighbor, then we went to friend's house in Winston Salem. It was Thanksgiving weekend, and when we came back Sunday evening to Durham, we stayed in the attic apartment of some friends for five days. Finally, we moved into the home of another family and rented out their basement space. The kids were 11 and 14 and they were extremely angry. We stayed that way for three years."

Still technically a dependent spouse and without legal authorization to work, Rajendra did not know how to pay for rent or food. The answer came quickly: cooking. Several years earlier, when her husband had been unemployed, Rajendra had cooked food for some neighbors in exchange for cash. The response was very positive: "My neighbors said 'Your food is so good, it is marketable, do this: cook for us and we'll come pick it up.' At first I was cooking for 27 people out of 12 homes, but the word slowly grew, and soon I was cooking 35–40 meals once a week. That was 160 meals a month, and I was charging $5 per meal." Rajendra's initial foray into cooking for a living ended in the face of her husband's rage, but upon returning to it after leaving him she found that she still had the skills needed to grow a business. "In that basement space, during those three years, we started Vimala's Take Out. I would buy all the produce that would be available for quick sale early in the morning, for 30 to 35 meals. Most of the time we would make just enough money for food to eat and rent. We had no child support, no permission to work, no alimony. As soon as my husband and I filed a separation agreement, my visa status expired to no status. I was underground for eleven years, from 1994 to 2005."

Using an email mailing list of more than 1500 names, Rajendra's take-out business grew rapidly out of the basement apartment. She and her food operation soon moved into a larger space, then resolved to expand to a formal commercial storefront.

"We got the key to our restaurant one March, and by the middle of May, served our first test meal. On May 31st we were wide open to the community. That's how we launched."

Opening the Restaurant

Rajendra's business opened in 2010, and that's when we discovered each other. I noticed that Curry Blossom Café was putting into practice so many of the employment standards that we call "taking the high road." The restaurant offers casual counter service, but there are both counter and credit-card tips, and there are workers who would traditionally be considered tipped employees, like Rajendra's two bartenders. Nevertheless, as Rajendra tells it, "at the Curryblossom Café, the minimum wage is $10 an hour plus tips. That was the minimum wage from the very beginning for the restaurant. None of this tipped minimum-wage business. After about a year, workers can receive a promotion and become a trainer of new employees. Some people are making $11, $12, or $13 an hour, plus tips on top of that. Most people can advance to $11 or $12 within a year. So with tips on top of that we're trying to approximate a living wage here in North Carolina."

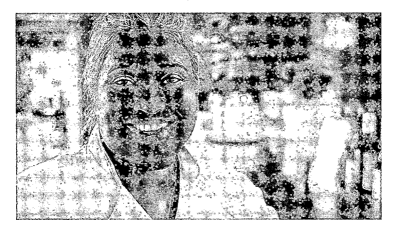

Vimala Rajendra.

When asked why she feels it is important to pay as close to a living wage as possible, Rajendra refers to her own experience. "I personally have worked for low wages as a babysitter when I didn't have a green card. I was making like $7 per hour. I did that for nine years. It's morally wrong to get work out of people who can't support their families. We wanted people to be able to make this a career, a livelihood."

"For me to say to Antonio, one of my prep cooks, 'Your prep is so good, you did a good job. You're my best worker. I'd pay you more if you spoke English." What good is that to me? Antonio's my highest paid employee. We pay him $900 per week. He has three daughters in elementary school. He's making more that $20 an hour."

Beyond wages, offering benefits is very important to Rajendra. Workers receive both paid vacation and paid sick days. "Some people don't take their vacation, so we just give them a check." Rajendra has also created her own form of health care for the workers: "We created a home grown primary healthcare plan. We have all these relationships with primary-care doctors—eye care specialists, general practitioners, dentists. It doesn't cost employees anything to get care. The company—Curryblossom Creations—pays each of the medical care providers a lump sum, like $1000 each year. Each time one of workers visits them, it chips away at that lump sum. We haven't dealt with a major medical problem, except for our Sous Chef, for whom we had to pay a $1500 medical bill."

However, other kinds of benefits are also important to Rajendra, especially childcare. "We have a single mother working in the restaurant. She's of Pakistani descent; she had never worked in a restaurant, but I hired her and said we would train her. As a single mom she had a hard time keeping all her hours. After working with us for six months, we discovered that, through an accounting error, we had been paying her $20 an hour instead of $10 an hour, for six months. We give tremendous leverage for single parents to be with their children, at home, during dinnertime. Sometimes we allow the caregiver to bring the child to the restaurant so the child can be near their parent. When we found out that she was being paid $20 an hour instead of $10, we said keep that. Instead of having her feel a tremendous paycut going back to $10 an hour, we told her we would give her a $100 childcare bonus per month to be added to her pay."

At that point, Rajendra decided to offer the same to all her employees. "We told all the employees, if you have a child, and you wish to take this, we will give you $100 childcare bonus per month. The workers understand we are not rolling in dough, but one guy asked us to pay for his 5-year-old's summer camp expenses, so we found an arrangement to pay for summer camp."

Why all these extras? "If you're invested in the community, you get social capital. You get enhanced benefits. Unlike big restaurant chains like the Olive Garden, we are rooted in our community. Even if we were to start a franchise, we'd tell the franchisee, 'Be rooted in the community. Build your own social capital. Our model can be replicated."

As for sexual harassment on the job, Rajendra learned from her father to espouse a culture of respect with her staff. "There is no place for any gender bias at the Curryblossom Café. I knew from my family and parents that a woman shouldn't be talked to in a certain way—but I also knew one thing deep inside, that a woman has the right and responsibility to intercept this kind of behavior. I tell all my women employees that this is a safe zone where there is zero tolerance for physical or sexual advances, verbally or nonverbally."

Olive Garden also claims a zero tolerance policy. So what makes Rajendra's zero tolerance policy different? "It's a woman-owned restaurant. Being a survivor of family violence, I'm someone who makes sure that abuse shouldn't go either way to anybody. There needs to be mutual respect in the workplace."

Rajendra feels strongly about her employees not having to tolerate any kind of inappropriate behavior from customers. "I'm very vocal about not putting our workers at [the] mercy of guests to be paid. By that I mean, the workers are there to work for me and with me and I should pay them. They are the employees of Curryblossom. They're not employed by the guests, therefore the guests shouldn't be paying the wages of my workers."

That's why, Rajendra says, she opposes the lower wage for tipped workers. "I'm absolutely against the tipped minimum wage of $2.13. How could this nation, calling itself a developed nation, stand around and talk about modern-day slavery elsewhere, when a waiter can be paid next to nothing? This is not fair. I've asked a lot of waiters, men and women, whether their employers are making up [the] difference [between the tipped minimum wage and the regular minimum wage]. The answer is always no. They say, 'We'd like to work only busy nights, but only certain people who make the cut get busy nights. If I'm working Monday nights I'm making very little or nothing at all.' I've asked waitresses when I eat out: 'You must be on this $2.13 an hour, does your employer inform you that you must earn the remainder in tips?' They draw a blank."

Rajendra hopes to expand to a full-service restaurant but would never pay the tipped minimum wage. "We hope to get a new place, a hybrid, where there's one counter-service casual section and one section [for] fine dining. The food is absolutely exquisite. People from different places, even Indians, and say it's the best Indian food. But even if we did fine dining, with sit-down service at dinnertime, our wait staff would be paid $10 minimum, or more."

Reporters often ask Rajendra how she manages to provide higher wages and benefits and make a profit. "I had a reporter in here the other day trying to get me to say how much profit I make. We're a single-family business, run by a woman who was a single mom for ten years. That being said, we made $650,000 in our first year, paying higher wages. We're making enough to pay off debts, live well, and create so many livelihoods. I have five employees who've only ever worked in restaurants. They've all said this was their best working environment ever. I asked them why, and they said, 'It's not all about the money. Here we feel valued, we feel respected.' "

Is Vimala's food more expensive because she pays livable wages? "It's a good idea to value the food enough, or the guests might think less of it. Our entrees are $14-$17 each. And it's good food. We've thought about raising the prices $1 here or $1 there. When we did that a few years ago, absolutely nobody noticed it. Manju [Rajendra's daughter] kept saying that the food had to be lower priced. One day I just walked in and changed all the prices on the menu. Manju never said anything, I don't think she ever even noticed it. The customers didn't either."

NOTES

1. Kerry Segrave, *Tipping: An American Social History of Gratuities.* (Jefferson, North Carolina: McFarland & Company, 1998), 9–43.
2. Ibid, 10, citing, John Gilmer Speed, "Tips and commissions," *Lippincott's Magazine* 69, 1902, p. 748.
3. Ibid, pp.11.
4. Ibid, pp.11, 52.
5. Ibid, p. 11.
6. Ibid, p. 61, citing "A No-Tip Hotel," *New York Times,* June 5, 1921, pt. 6, p. 7; "Scientific tipping," *New York Times,* September 3, 1922, pt. 6, p. 8.
7. Ibid. p. 61, citing Will Payne, "Tips," *Saturday Evening Post* 198, 1926, pp. 33, 86.
8. 29 U.S.C., § 8 (1938).
9. Pub. L. No. 89–601, §101(a) (1966).
10. David H. Bradley. "The Tip Credit Provisions of the Fair Labor Standards Act (FLSA): In Brief." *Congressional Research Service* 7–5700, R43445, March 27, 2014. < https://www.hsdl.org/?view&did=752100>.
11. Restaurant Opportunities Centers United (ROC United), et al., *The Other NRA: Unmasking the Agenda of the National Restaurant Association.* (New York, NY: Restaurant Opportunities Centers United, 2014).

12. Sylvia Allegretto and David Cooper. "Twenty-Three Years and Still Waiting for Change: Why It's Time to Give Tipped Workers the Regular Minimum Wage." *Economic Policy Institute*. N.p., July 10, 2014. <http://www.epi.org/publication/waiting-for-change-tipped-minimum-wage/>.

13. "Minimum Wages for Tipped Employees," Wage and Hour Division (WHD, U.S. Department of Labor, January 1, 2015, http://www.dol.gov/whd/state/tipped.htm.

14. Dave Jamieson, "Herman Cain's Distrust of Minimum Wage Goes Back to His Restaurant Days," *The Huffington Post*, October 27, 2011. <http://www.huffingtonpost.com/2011/10/27/herman-cain-minimum-wage_n_1035157.html>.

15. "Majority of states reject minimum wage increases,", *National Restaurant Association*, June 3, 2013. <http://www.restaurant.org/News-Research/News/Majority-of-states-reject-minimum-wage-increases>.

16. ROC United, *Recipe for Success: Abolish the Subminimum Wage* (New York, NY: ROC United, 2014).

17. Roberto Ferdman, "Which US States Tip the Most (and Least), as Shown by Millions of Square transactions," *Quartz*, March 21, 2014, http://qz.com/189458/the-united-states-of-tipping/.

18. Ibid.

19. Alan Greenblatt, "After 23 Years, Your Waiter Is Ready For A Raise." *NPR*. Feb. 11, 2014, <http://www.npr.org/blogs/thesalt/2014/02/06/272469496/after-23-years-your-waiter-is-ready-for-a-raise>.

20. "Employment and Wages for the Highest and Lowest Paying Occupations, May 2014." *US Bureau of Labor Statistics*. n.p., 2013. http://www.bls.gov/oes/2014/may/high_low_paying.htm.

21. ROC United, Family Values @ Work, HERvotes Coalition, et al., *Tipped Over the Edge: Gender Inequity in the Restaurant Industry* (New York, NY: Restaurant Opportunities Centers United, 2012).

22. ROC United, *Picking Up the NRA's Tab: The Public Cost of Low Wages in the Restaurant Industry* (New York, NY: Restaurant Opportunities Centers United, 2015).

23. Restaurant Opportunities Centers United & Forward Together, October 7th, 2014. *The Glass Floor: Sexual Harassment in the Restaurant Industry*. (New York, NY: Restaurant Opportunities Centers United).

24. Restaurant Opportunities Centers United & Forward Together, *The Glass Floor: Sexual Harassment in the Restaurant Industry*. (New York, NY: Restaurant Opportunities Centers United, 2014).

25. To Come

26. "Tipping in Italy." *Guidelines for Tipping in Italy*. n.p., 2013, http://tours-italy.com/italy-tourism/travel-guide/tipping/; "Italy: How to Fit in with the Locals." - *TripAdvisor*. n.p., Dec. 10, 2014. <http://www.

tripadvisor.com/Travel-g187768-c2815/Italy:How.To.Fit.In.With. The.Locals.html>.

27. Darden Restaurants, Inc. "Company Profile, Information, Business Description, History, Background Information on Darden Restaurants, Inc.," http://www.referenceforbusiness.com/history2/73/Darden-Restaurants-Inc.html (accessed 23 February 2015).

28. Philip Mattera and Thomas Mattera. "Corporate Research Rap Sheet: Darden Restaurants," Good Jobs First, 2015. Updated October 13, 2014. http://www.corp-research.org/darden

29. Annual Report. "Darden Restaurants Inc." *Darden*, July 18, 2014. <http://investor.darden.com/files/doc_financials/071814-10k_v001_x2ipxc.pdf>

30. Ibid.

31. Ibid.

32. Lowrey, Annie. "Olive Garden Has Middle-Class Problem." *Daily Intelligencer*, September 17, 2014. <http://nymag.com/daily/intelligencer/2014/09/olive-garden-has-middle-class-problems.html>.

33. Brad Tuttle, "Olive Garden Admits Making Up 'Authentic' Italian Dishes Like Pastachetti." *TIME*, July 12, 2011. http://business.time.com/2011/07/12/olive-garden-admits-making-up-authentic-italian-dishes-like-pastachetti/>.

34. The Associated Press. "Profit Declines for Owner of Olive Garden." *The New York Times*, June 20, 2014, < http://www.nytimes.com/2014/06/21/business/profit-declines-for-owner-of-olive-garden.html?_r=0>.

35. Paul Brinkmann, "Olive Garden Update: How Designers Tackled the Job." *OrlandoSentinel.com*. n.p., July 29, 2014, <http://www.orlandosentinel.com/business/brinkmann-on-business/os-olive-garden-update-how-designers-tackled-the-job-20140729-post.html>.

36. "Transforming Darden Restaurants." *Starboard Value*, September 11, 2014. <http://www.documentcloud.org/documents/1300752-transforming-darden.html>

37. Ashley Lutz, "This Map Shows How Your State Feels About Olive Garden." *Business Insider*, <http://www.businessinsider.com/olive-garden-america-yelp-rating-map-2014-9>.

38. "Transforming Darden Restaurants." *Starboard Value*, September 11, 2014. <http://www.documentcloud.org/documents/1300752-transforming-darden.html>.

39. Ibid., 114-125.

40. Ibid., 116.

41. Pyke, Alan. "Olive Garden Illustrated Corporate America's Worst Financial Tendencies," *Thinkprogress.org*, October 6, 2014. <http://thinkprogress.org/economy/2014/10/06/3576521/olive-garden-darden-parachute-share holders/>.

42. Sarah Anderson, "Darden's Golden Goodbyes," *Institute for Policy Studies*, October 1, 2014, < http://www.ips-dc.org/wp-content/uploads/2014/10/Darden-executive-retirement-packages.pdf >.

43. Lisa Jennings, "Darden Defends Pay Practices," *Nation's Restaurant News*, September 25, 2013, http://m.nrn.com/casual-dining/darden-defends-pay-practices?page=2.

44. Ibid.

45. "Norovirus is the leading cause of disease outbreaks from contaminated food in the US," Centers for Disease Control and Prevention, June 3, 2014. http://www.cdc.gov/media/releases/2014/p0603-norovirus.html>; Centers for Disease Control and Prevention, "Preventing Norovirus Outbreaks: Food service has a key role." *CDC Vitalsigns*, June 2014. http://www.cdc.gov/vitalsigns/pdf/2014-06-vitalsigns.pdf.

46. The New York Times, "Illnesses Close Restaurant," *The New York Times*, December 15, 2006, http://www.nytimes.com/2006/12/16/us/16olive.html?_r=0.

47. Chris Proffitt, "Health Dept.: Norovirus caused Olive Garden outbreak," *13WTHR.com Eyewitness News*, December 18, 2006, http://www.wthr.com/global/story.asp?S=5828920.

48. Philip Mattera, and Thomas Mattera. "Corporate Research Rap Sheet: Darden Restaurants," http://www.corp-research.org/darden, October 13, 2014.

49. Catharine Gensel, "Settlement in Hepatitis A Class Action in North Carolina," *NoroCORE Food Virology*, NCSU, October 18, 2012. http://norocore.ncsu.edu/settlement-in-hepatitis-a-class-action-in-north-carolina/; Sarah Klein and Ray Hainer, "Olive Garden Diners in North Carolina Exposed to Hepatitis A," *Health Magazine*, August 10, 2011. < http://news.health.com/2011/08/10/hepatitis-olive-garden/>

50. "Olive Garden Settles Indiana Suit over Norovirus Contamination." *Class Action Reporter*, 10, no. 246, December 11, 2008, http://bankrupt.com/CAR_Public/081211.mbx
Corporate Research Rap Sheet: Darden Restaurants.

51. http://articles.latimes.com/2011/sep/15/news/la-pn-michelle-obama-menu-20110915.

52. Ibid.

53. "Darden Settles More Wage & Hour Class Actions." *Wage Law*, January 11, 2008, http://www.californiawagelaw.com/wage_law/2008/01/darden-settles.html

54. "Darden Settles Ex-worker's Lawsuit in California," *Orlando Sentinel*, July 18, 2008, <http://articles.orlandosentinel.com/2008-07-18/news/c3report18_1_olive-garden-darden-asus>.

55. DOL News Brief, "Texas Restaurant Chain Agrees to Pay Back Wages, Civil Penalties," *United States Department of Labor*, April 14, 2011. http://www.dol.gov/_sec/newsletter/2011/20110414.htm>.

56. Curt Anderson, "Olive Garden, LongHorn Workers Sue Company Alleging Wage Violations," *Huffington Post*, September 7, 2012, http://www.huffingtonpost.com/2012/09/07/olive-garden-lawsuit_n_1864042.html; Mattera, Philip & Thomas Mattera. Corporate Research Rap Sheet: Darden Restaurants, October 13, 2014, http://www.corp-research.org/darden.

57. Sandra Pedicini, "Darden Restaurants enforces tip-sharing policy," *Orlando Sentinel*, February 10, 2011. < http://articles.orlandosentinel.com/2011-02-10/business/os-darden-employees-pay-20110210_1_darden-restaurants-bartenders-tip-sharing>; Candace Choi and Ricardo Alonso-Zaldivar, "Darden Restaurants Test Hiring of More Part-Time Employees to Avoid Obamacare Costs." *Huffington Post*, October 09, 2012, <http://www.huffingtonpost.com/2012/10/09/darden- restaurants-obamacare-part-time_n_1951103.html>.

58. Yuki Noguchi,. "As Health Law Changes Loom, A Shift to Part-Time Workers." *NPR*, April 29, 2013, <http://www.npr.org/2013/04/29/179864601/as-health-law-changes-loom-a-shift-to-part-time-workers>.

59. *Wilson v. Darden Restaurants, Inc.*, No. CIV. A. 99-5020, 2000 WL 150872, at *1 (E.D. Pa. Feb. 11, 2000), < https://casetext.com/case/wilson-v-darden-restaurants-inc>.

60. *Baier v. Darden Restaurants*, 420 S.W.3d 733 (Mo. Ct. App. 2014).

61. Sandra Pedicini, "Al Sharpton's Group Urges Big Investors to Drop Darden Stock." *Orlando Sentinel*, February 1, 2011, http://articles.orlandosentinel.com/2011-02-01/business/os-darden-sharpton-complaints-20110131_1_smokey-bones-darden-restaurants-bahama-breeze-restaurant>.

62. Ibid.

[3]

FINE DINING

The Great Service Divide

The growth of the fine dining sector over the last two decades has given rise to the term "foodie," a now-ubiquitous moniker applied to individuals who celebrate and seek out the finer and more-rare sections of the food-service spectrum. With fine dining now one of the fastest growing segments of the restaurant industry, celebrity-chef-owned restaurants have become all the rage. Although the total number of workers in casual restaurants remains much larger, fine dining and fast food have been growing more rapidly than the casual restaurants in the middle,[1] perhaps a reflection of growing income inequality in America. In spite of the recent recession, American consumers have demonstrated a willingness to pay more for what they perceive as higher-quality food and service they believe they can obtain at a fine dining restaurant.

Unfortunately, even though menu prices might be higher in fine dining restaurants, it has not necessarily translated into higher wages and benefits for workers. See Table 3.1.

Of course, there are a few notable standouts. Several of our high-road employer partners fall into the fine dining category and fare quite well on raises, benefits, and promotions. Two in particular— Tom Colicchio and Andy Shallal—intentionally work to overcome the typical race and gender segregation in the fine dining segment. See Table 3.2.

Table 3.2 LOW-ROAD RESTAURANTS

	$10+ Wage for Non-Tipped Workers	Hourly Wage for Tipped Workers Exceeds Minimum	Paid Sick Days?	Promotion Practices?	Stars
Del Frisco's Steak House					
Fleming's Prime Steakhouse and Wine Bar		$+			
Fogo de Chão					
Morton's The Steakhouse					
Ruth's Chris Steak House					
Shula's Steak House					
Texas de Brazil Churrascaria					
The Capital Grille					
The Melting Pot					
The Palm					

Table 3.1 HIGH-ROAD RESTAURANTS

	$10+ Wage for Non-Tipped Workers	Hourly Wage for Tipped Workers Exceeds Minimum	Paid Sick Days?	Promotion Practices?	Stars
Craft Los Angeles *Los Angeles, CA*	💵	💲+		←	★★
Eatonville *Washington, DC*			🌡	←	★
Gramercy Tavern *New York, NY*	💵	n/a*		←	★★
iCi *Brooklyn, NY*	💵		🌡	←	★★
Killen's Steakhouse *Pearland, TX*	💵		🌡	←	★★
One if by Land, Two if by Sea *New York, NY*	💵		🌡	←	★★
Red Hill Restaurant *Los Angeles, CA*	💵	💲+	🌡	←	★★
The Modern *New York, NY*	💵	n/a*		←	★★
Union Square Café *New York, NY*	💵	n/a*		←	★★

*No tipped employees

The price divide between fine dining restaurants and other restaurant segments has opened the door to additional inequities, specifically those related to pay, race, and gender segregation. Based on price points alone, it is not surprising that that servers and bartenders in fine dining restaurants can earn so much more than their counterparts in casual restaurants. It has also created more severe occupational segregation and discrimination by race and gender in fine dining restaurants than in any other segment of the industry.

In 2014, ROC released a series of reports called "The Great Service Divide," based on matched-pairs audit-testing studies conducted in New York, Chicago, Detroit, and New Orleans. Working with the foremost employment discrimination expert in the country, Mark Bendick, ROC sent white and people-of-color applicants, with identical resumes and body types, to apply for fine dining server positions. A tremendous amount of time and capital was committed to training these white and people-of-color applicants to mimic one another's mannerisms and personality types, all to ensure that the only palpable difference between the candidates was their race. The results were stark: in larger cities, white applicants were twice as likely to obtain livable-wage fine dining server positions as people of color, even when the people of color had better resumes. White applicants were treated better by management and given more time to speak and interview. This kind of discrimination has resulted in a $4 per hour wage gap between white workers and workers of color in the restaurant industry nationwide.[2] The percentage of workers of color in fine dining waitstaff and bartending positions is less than half the percentage of workers of color in the industry overall.[3]

There are a handful of restaurant owners working to overcome racial segregation in the industry. One is Andy Shallal, owner of the Busboys and Poets restaurant group in Washington, DC and the surrounding region. An immigrant from Iraq, Shallal has been involved in social-justice activities since his youth.

As an adult working as a server in a restaurant, Shallal was struck by the unfair and capricious nature of working for tips. "It feels very demeaning for a professional. It sends the message, 'I'm not worthy, and I beg you to give me whatever you can.'" The inverse of this relationship, Shallal argues, is that customers can exercise dissatisfaction by withholding gratuity—thereby making sure a server doesn't get paid. "It's one thing to say someone didn't do a good job; you can call a manager to say that. But the manager has no right to tell the worker, 'you didn't do a good job, so I'm not going to pay you today,'" Shallal says. "As the customer, you're actually allowed to not pay someone if they don't please you. The fact that the restaurant is supposed to make up the difference if someone doesn't like a server—that's psychologically strange."

In 2005 Shallal opened Busboys and Poets, the combination bookstore, event space, and restaurant that has both made him famous and come to embody his political views. The eight locations in three states employ more than 600 people, and all are committed to paying livable wages and maintaining a culture of diversity and social justice.

Shallal's greatest tool in fostering this culture is hiring all types of people and then promoting them. "I'm always thinking about diversity—not having too many of one kind of person in any position. Lots of places have an intense divide between the front of the house staff and the back of the house. But if you have people of different backgrounds in both, it helps with the interaction between front and back. It creates bridges all around." Shallal says it isn't always easy. "You have to be very intentional about it. There are times when I'll glance at the staff and notice that there is a concentration of one group or another in a position. I'll tell the manager—'Are you aware of it?' You have to change processes to make up for inadequacies that are glaring."

Engineering racial diversity isn't always easy, and it isn't always what diners think they want: "People want to see people who look like them serving them." However, the upshot of going against this grain is mutual enlightenment. "People with different backgrounds have different styles. That's the exciting thing about being [a] server—being able to experience different cultures."

Being intentional about diversity in the workplace makes Shallal's restaurants unique in the industry. He identifies it as his core mission. "It is part of our tribal statement—we consciously uplift racial, cultural connections. That doesn't just apply to customers, that applies to our own group. How do we create those connections?"

In addition to immersion, Shallal encourages these connections through an upfront conversation about race and identity. At the same time that new employees are brought in for training and orientation, they are also brought in to a group conversation about race and culture. "We ask them how race impacts their lives," Shallal says. "We ask them to share racial and cultural experiences they've had—the positives and the negatives. Every two weeks, I spend three hours with a new group of people coming in. It's a very intense, very emotional experience. Every time I've done it, there's crying and catharsis."

Shallal acknowledges that some employees leave after the meeting and don't return; such is the necessary attrition that comes with progress. "Race is one of those things we don't like to talk about, something we can't ignore. The conversation is deep, honest, and rich. By the end of the session, we become very close."

What may be difficult aspects of this initial immersion in the Busboys and Poets culture gives way quickly to a working culture that is reflective of the diverse city in which the business is situated.

"In a space of intentionality—where there are different types of people—it makes for a much richer experience, more representative of city I live in. I want to make sure that experience doesn't get watered down. Some employers might say 'this is too much of a headache, let's just make money.' For me, if I make intentional diversity the focus, everybody will understand. They won't just be words on paper. I decided that this is something I have to commit to. If nothing else, this is the number one thing."

THE HIGH ROAD: THE CRAFT OF PROMOTING FROM WITHIN

Tom Colicchio, celebrity chef star of Bravo's *Top Chef* series, grew up in working-class New Jersey, the son of a correction officer in a county jail. As a union member, Tom's father would talk to him about working conditions on the job, and about politicians who did not seem to care about taking care of people. "He was always sticking up for the underdog."

Colicchio learned to cook as a teenager by watching his mother in her kitchen. But Tom also started working in restaurants around the same age. "I started my first restaurant job at the age of 15 at a seafood restaurant in Elizabeth, New Jersey. I was a busser, and I earned $2 an hour plus tips." Asked to describe the tipping culture for bussers like him, Colicchio says, "The waiters would just give me whatever tips they wanted to give me."

Colicchio's work diversified when he graduated from high school at age 17. "I was constantly being asked to do things that I wasn't paid to do. 'Go drive a truck to our sister restaurant, but first go punch out,' they'd say. I'd routinely work 70 to 80 hours per week." One of the places he worked, a family-style Italian restaurant, offered Colicchio and other workers "shift pay," a common (and highly illegal) practice in which management pays employees a lump sum for a shift of indeterminate length. "They'd just pay you a certain amount for the shift, and you'd work and work. You'd just go home whenever you go home – no hourly wage, no overtime." Another restaurant paid Colicchio a salary when he should have been paid as an hourly work, and had him work 80 hours a week with no overtime.

Colicchio quickly ascended the ranks, working in many of New York City's restaurants and landing as executive chef at the restaurant Mondrian by age 26. His work at Mondrian quickly attracted praise, including a three-star review from the *New York Times* and being named one of the city's "best new chefs" by *Food &Wine.*

All this experience served to inform Colicchio's approach to the business. "I always said, 'When I get my own restaurant, I'm going to do things differently.' Fortunately, when the time came to open my own first restaurant, I partnered with a guy who felt exactly the same way."

Opening the First Restaurant

Colicchio's favorable reception wasn't limited to critics. Another admirer was Danny Meyer, a new and respected restaurateur known for his wildly successful Union Square Café. "I knew he liked what I was doing. Danny and his wife would come to Mondrian to eat. Other people from Union Square would come." The critical praise elicited by Colicchio's work as a chef often landed him at events with Meyer, including the 1993 Food & Wine Classic in Aspen. There, Colicchio made his approach. "I told him, 'I think you like what I do. Why don't we open a place together?' Danny said he wasn't interested in opening a second restaurant. But a week later he called back saying he wanted to do it. He told me later that a friend had told him, 'If Sandy Koufax wanted to pitch for your team, you'd say yes.' So he said yes."

Colicchio and Meyer traveled to Italy together to brainstorm ideas and concepts for the new venture. Trips like this are common among chefs; what was uncommon about this one was what they discussed. "We didn't talk about the food. We talked all about what kind of restaurant we wanted to open – what kind of conditions we wanted to create for workers, what kind of ambience. We saw eye to eye. I think that was Danny's way of interviewing me, making sure he knew I was on board with the way he ran his business. It was all about taking care of employees first—pay people fairly, and they'll take care of you. He had no idea that those were already my ideas. I had found a complete ally."

Colicchio and Meyer opened Gramercy Tavern together in 1994. "When we opened, we put it all into practice. Above all else, it was about treating people fairly. We made sure they were getting schedules ahead of time. We gave people time off. We were non-smoking before the smoking ban. Besides the fact that both of our fathers had died of cancer, we thought, 'Why are we forcing our employees to sit through cigarette smoke?' It was all about treating people with respect and dignity. We always talked about legitimizing the restaurant business—being professional, being open. We'd sit down with the employees and talk about the profit and loss statements."

Colicchio made sure to take care of his staff in ways that he himself had not been taken care of—and in ways that are fairly unheard of in the restaurant industry. "We evaluated the waitstaff every year to give them a raise. I remember throwing someone out of the restaurant for disrespecting a server. I was in the kitchen, and someone came and told me that a guest had said to a female server, 'Fat waitress—get away from me!' I went straight over to the customer and asked him if he had said it." When the customer did not deny that he made the comment, Colicchio asked him to leave immediately. "He tried to come back to the restaurant on other days with other people's names on the reservation. But I never let him back in the restaurant." On another occasion, he refused a regular's request to bring a stripper to a party. "I said no way. I knew it wouldn't sit well with half my employees."

In the kitchen, all workers earned more than the minimum wage, and yearly evaluations resulted in annual raises. "It was all about promoting people, letting people know that there was a path to becoming a sous chef, path to grow. If there were [bussers] who wanted to become waiters but couldn't speak English well, we brought in a teacher to teach them English. There was never a question of how much we'd have to spend—it was critical to invest in our employees. Because above all, we knew that someone who started as a [busser] and is now a captain would be fully invested in what we're doing."

Providing Opportunities

Promotion from within and internal raises and promotions has been a fundamental tenet of Colicchio's that has carried over from Gramercy Tavern into the restaurants he now owns on his own. "At one point [a consultant] came in and said, 'You're paying people a lot of money—you should throw them out and hire newer people whom you can pay less.' I said no way. I know the quality of work I get out of them—it's so good, it's as good as two new people."

In 2001, with Gramercy Tavern firmly rooted among New York's best restaurants, Colicchio sold his shares to Meyer and opened his own restaurant, Craft, one block away. At Craft, Colicchio implemented all the same above-average wages, benefits, and promotions practices. "Wages are important, but it's just as important for you to know that you can grow and make more money, that there is upward mobility, that you can start here, and end up in a better place."

As praise for Craft piled up and Colicchio's team of employees grew, he needed to provide more positions for people to grow into. "We never looked at opportunities to grow as [being] about 'how big can we get?'" It's more about providing new opporunities to people within the restaurant. I have a porter who became a garde-manger, a line cook, and now he is a sous chef. Having more restaurants provides more opportunities to people, so they don't max out. You have cooks who want to be sous chefs, starting managers who wanted to become general managers. How to provide all these opportunities for people to grow? Grow the business."

As Colicchio's brand of Craft restaurants has grown across locations and cities—three in New York, with additional locations in Las Vegas and Los Angeles–each restaurant continues to provide above-average wages and benefits to workers. Everyone is offered health benefits, and the restaurant pays a portion for anyone who opts in. All workers receive vacation time after their first year of work. "We provided paid sick days before it became the law in New York."

But what makes Craft especially unique, even among other very fine dining restaurants, is the racial diversity of the serving staff and management. Colicchio attributes this to the company's commitment to promote from within. "We've had lots of workers move from [busser] to waiter to captain. It's because they deserve it. If you're ready, if you want it, it's yours for the taking. If you need to learn better English, we'll teach you better English. If they deserve it, they're going to get that shot."

Promoting from within means that workers of color who start in lower-level positions end up in server, bartender, captain, and management positions on the dining floor. Perhaps as a result, Craft has a reputation of being a good place to work for people of color.

"We don't consciously hire a certain kind of person. But perhaps it's the way we treat people, from the top all the way down. I don't know what makes someone stay and want a promotion. Perhaps it's just the fact that we're making people feel comfortable so they stick around. Perhaps it's the fact that our staff members refer their friends to work here." When there's an opening at any of the Craft restaurants, the policy is to always inform all the staff in all the various restaurants first. "We almost never have an opening in a higher level position that we can't fill internally. We're always looking for talent. We tell a [busser]: 'This server position might open up; come in early, watch the other servers. Watch how they pour the wine. Pay more attention.'"

Every day, the company has all the waiters and bussers try a new wine. "During family meal, everyone is taught about a new wine. They learn about the taste and the color and the feel." Wine training for lower-level staff is unique, and it sometimes means that immigrant workers with accents ascend from less visible jobs to servers. "Sometimes you hear a customer say, 'I don't understand this person. Give me someone who speaks better English.' It depends on the situation. If the person is genuinely having a hard time understanding, we might try to help. But if the person is just being nasty, we'll say, 'This person understands the menu, and is qualified to be here. This is your waiter.' They have people with very strong French accents in French restaurants; why can't workers with other accents be waiters?"

Tipped Over the Edge

Colicchio is aware of recent research that indicates that tipping is quite often not a reflection of service, but rather correlated with unconscious biases. "I went to an event where a neuroscientist was presenting on [a concept called] the 'light touch': They said that if a male server lightly touches a guest, the server will get a worse tip. If a female server lightly touches a guest, she will get a better tip, from both men and women."

"I would be in favor of getting rid of tips altogether, and paying waiters a livable wage. At my restaurant that would mean $28-$30 an hour." As of September 2015, Colicchio has started to do just that, eliminating tipping at lunchtime in one of his restaurants. One month later, and after several months of discussions with ROC that included an address to the Union Square Hospitality Group staff on the history and social impact of the tipped minimum wage, Danny Meyer announced that he would also move to eliminate tipping in his restaurants.

There is another reason Colicchio favors eliminating the lower wage for tipped workers: it creates tremendous liability for employers. The tipped minimum wage is a complicated and antiquated law that requires employers to ensure that tips make up the difference between the lower minimum wage for tipped workers and the regular minimum wage. In New York State, there are additional burdens that require employers to inform every new employee that they are being paid the lower tipped minimum wage, and that tips will make up the difference, and even a requirement to officially notify workers when they are receiving a raise.[4] As a result, several employment attorneys have developed whole practices suing employers like Colicchio for violating these complicated tipping laws. "There's a whole cottage industry of attorneys who are making their living off this two-tiered system. Some of the cases are merited; many are not. They can get someone on a technicality about whether they sent out a notice of a raise. It's absolutely wrong. Do I think someone taking tips from servers to pay managers should be punished? Absolutely. But some of these attorneys are acting in their own self-interest. If we got rid of the lower minimum wage for tipped workers, that would go away."

THE LOW ROAD: THE CAPITAL GRILLE

The Capital Grille was founded by Edward Grace III in Providence Rhode Island in 1990.[5] The brand was acquired by Darden Restaurants in 2007. Today there are 54 locations centered in major metropolitan areas.[6] The Capital Grille stands as Darden's most upscale brand, with an average check of $72 per person, compared with $16.75 per person at Olive Garden. It is also one of Darden's more successful chains, with same-restaurant sales increase of 3.4 percent in financial 2014 over the previous year.[7]

Upon its founding by Grace, The Capital Grille elicited praise from the critical community, including a 1996 "Hot Concept" award from Nation's Restaurant News and a "Best Award of Excellence" from Wine Spectator. With this success, Grace rose to chairman of government relations at the National Restaurant Association in 1996 and has been a director of Boston Restaurant Associates Inc. since April 2004.

The company takes great pride in its food and beverage quality. "The Capital Grille has locations in metropolitan cities in the United States. The Capital Grille offers seafood flown in daily and culinary specials created by its chefs. The restaurants feature a wine list offering over 350 selections, personalized service, and private dining rooms."[8]The Capital Grille is Darden's most upscale chain, cultivating a fine dining experience with the strongest reception among Darden concepts in dining publications that issue awards and accolades.[9] The Capital Grille has thrived during the recession, largely because of its more affluent customer base.[10]

Workers Speak Up

In 2012, with assistance from ROC, workers in five states filed lawsuits against The Capital Grille alleging racial discrimination and wage violations. The lawsuits alleged that the company favored white workers over people of color for lucrative tipped jobs, and that they required tipped workers to share their earnings with nontipped workers.[11] By January of 2014, almost 20,000 former and current Darden Restaurant workers joined the suit.[12] However, due to an earlier Supreme Court ruling prohibiting class action lawsuits of this kind, in September 2014, a Federal District Court Judge decertified the class and held that servers could file individual lawsuits against the company.[13]

In 2013, employees at a Pittsburgh Capital Grille location—and members of ROC—protested having to work on Thanksgiving without holiday pay.[14] Following this, Pittsburgh City Council passed a Will of Council measure opposing the restaurant's decision to force employees to work on Thanksgiving without holiday pay.[15]

Horacio's Story at The Capital Grille

Horacio was born in Mexico City, the eighth of nine children. "We grew up very poor. I remember when I was 5 or 6 years old, going to the market. There were big trucks of oranges and beans. My dad used to take me there, and we used to help unload the trucks. My dad used to tell me to go to the driver and ask him, 'Can you let me sweep the truck?' In that way we used to recover pounds of beans and corn. We'd take that home and eat that."

Horacio's parents worked as bathroom attendants in the same public market in Mexico City. As the children in the family graduated high school, they began leaving for the States one by one in search of higher-paying jobs. In 1993, amid rampant inflation stemming from the devaluation of the peso, Horacio became the third male of his family to leave for the states, following two brothers who had landed and found work at a Chinese restaurant. His journey from Mexico City to Pittsburgh was harrowing: After flying from Mexico City to Tijuana, he and a friend crossed the border on foot. "It was 10 hours of running. There were ladies with kids; it was rough, but we made it." Horacio traveled from San Ysidro to San Diego and eventually Los Angeles, where he bought a one-way ticket to Pittsburgh. "It was 1993; back then you could take an airplane without a U.S. I.D."

The shock of cold and snow that greeted him in Pittsburgh was accompanied by a daily take-home pay between $20 and $25 as a busser and dishwasher at the Chinese restaurant. He remained resolute, quickly learning English and working as many hours as he could manage.

An Opportunity to Lead

Within a few months, Horacio was presented with an opportunity at another restaurant, this one more a more upscale establishment offering Spanish fare. Horacio was offered a busser position and an opportunity to do front-of-house work—rare for immigrants and persons of color—at a restaurant with considerably higher price points. The prices on the menu did not translate into higher pay for workers like Horacio, as the restaurant employed the pervasive "tip share" system for bussers. "I had never really worked in fine dining or any other restaurant besides the Chinese place. I had no clue about tip share, and the Spanish and Portuguese restaurants had the worst system I'd ever see in all my later years in the industry." The Spanish restaurant required all bussers to pool their tips, and they'd receive a percentage of the tips based on a complicated and arguably illegal system.

Horacio rose to server within two years, where he remained for an additional six years before moving with the company to Cincinnati, and later Cleveland, in managerial capacities. "I ran the place in Cleveland for about three years. We won all the awards – 'Best in the city,'

'Best service,' 'Best fine dining.'" Having worked for nearly a decade to become a general manager, he found himself unsatisfied, and conveyed as much to the ownership group. "After that, I told them 'Listen, I want to run a place where I can be a part owner.'"

Such a proclamation from Horacio was bold: he was still not a permanent resident of the United States, and had only recently received a work permit (via sponsorship of his employer) to work legally in the states. Ultimately the restaurant owners would leverage this to their advantage. "I helped them open another restaurant in Cleveland, and they promised me 10 percent of the partnership based on sweat equity. But after I opened the restaurant and was there for a year, they never gave me the documents to make it official." The partners continued the gambit by promising Horacio a larger ownership share if he opened another restaurant, this time back in Pittsburgh. "So I moved to Pittsburgh again. I created the first Spanish tapas restaurant in the city. I created the menu, designed everything myself." The restaurant opened to great success, and the owners continued to drag their feet. "They told me I needed a green card to be a partner, to be named on the business and the liquor license."

Horacio's determination was greater than his frustration, and he managed the Pittsburgh tapas restaurant to continued success while also abandoning the unfair wage practices that had been standard in his experience as a restaurant workers. "This was going to be *my* restaurant. I thought, 'I'm going to be more fair.'" In his equitable model, both servers and bussers made transparent and equitable shares of the tips.

After one year, Horacio revisited the issue of formalizing his share of ownership of the new restaurants, citing the company's 60 percent profit margin and increasing revenues across the twelve months. It was then that the partners informed him that he would not be an owner, nor would he continue as general manager. "They said, 'We're going to take over from here." Horacio was handed a check for $20,000—thanks for the "sweat equity" he had put in rather than general-manager-level salary—and asked to leave.

Horacio was furious and devastated. The "sweat equity" agreement had come as justification for a one-half reduction in his salary, and the proposed $20,000 didn't approach what he'd put into the business. "I was working 80 hours per week. I lost all the hours I worked, all the effort I put in. It was a shot to my heart. That place was my baby." Out of spite, and to his own detriment, Horacio didn't cash the $20,000 check.

"I cut it in a thousand pieces."

Starting at the Capital Grille

The Capital Grille opened in Pittsburgh around the time that Horacio's restaurant ownership dissolved. After the devastation of losing what he thought was to be his own business, Horacio resigned himself to serving rather than managing. "I was still broken hearted, and I was never able to put the money together to open my own place."

Upon arriving for his interview at Capital Grille, Horacio was put through a series of interviews with three different managers—more than usual for a server position, and more than his fellow applicants. He was hired as a server and, upon starting work at the restaurant, he observed a dynamic that may have contributed to a rather extensive vetting process. "There were only two Black servers there, and two Latinos—just me and this white-skinned Puerto Rican. I'm lighter skinned, so that probably helped me. There were no dark skinned Latinos."

Horacio continued to observe and experience racial injustices at the Capital Grille, in particular a ceiling for workers of color. Even Horacio, who was an observable exception to the culture in that he was allowed to serve, felt a cap on his advancement: he was not asked to train white employees. "It was me and four other servers who were supposed to train other people. After eight years, I told my boss, 'How come all these years, I'm only training Mexican and Portuguese workers? I think there's something wrong here, how you've got me categorized.'" The manager denied making any such distinction, but the trends persisted.

The employees that Horacio was allowed to train were uniformly Latino and uniformly relegated to bussing tables. "I trained two Latino servers. One of them was really good. I officially trained him, and he passed all his [server] tests. But they wouldn't put him as a server; they made him a busser and food runner." At the same time, a new, white server with less experience was hired and immediately put on the dining room floor as a server.

Both Horacio and the passed-over busser escalated their claims of discrimination to management; the busser suffered retaliation from the staff. "He went to his car, and they'd put this [note] in his dashboard: '*Stay where you belong, we have enough Latino servers.*'" (Note that their total number of Latino servers was holding steady at one: Horacio.)

As the protests from Horacio and the other Latino employee persisted, so, too, did the notes. Management's promises of change—giving the passed-over employee service shifts, making announcements reinforcing a company policy against harassment—never materialized. The frustrated employee left the restaurant for a different job.

According to Horacio, Capital Grille management acted quickly to avoid lingering appearances of discrimination. "Within weeks, they found this other Mexican guy to be a server. They let him become as server as soon as the training finished. They didn't mess with him as much."

Horacio was asked to train the Mexican server, which he did, but thereafter declined to train any additional employees. When pressed by management to reconsider, they offered to send him to other locations to train employees, too. The locations they proposed were in Mexico.

If there's any question about whether a person of color, or a person with a non-European accent, can make a good fine dining server, Horacio cites his customers' documented satisfaction as evidence to the contrary. "I have more guests who ask for me to serve them than anyone else in the restaurant: 600 guests regularly ask for me. The server with the next best record has 100. Most people have only five or ten guests who regularly ask for them; I have two or three tables every day." The systems that might conspire to hold him back are overmatched by his service ability. "That's what saved me, despite my skin color: These guests have my cell phone [number]. If I'm not there, they don't want to come."

Horacio still dreams of opening up his own restaurant. "This is giving me more incentive to do it myself. If I had my own place I'd be fair with everybody. It makes me mad to see a multimillion dollar company that doesn't split the wealth. I was raised like that. You don't just keep everything for you."

NOTES

1. Mark Brandau, "Fine Dining Traffic Growth Outpaces Other Segments," *Nation's Restaurant News*, April 8, 2014, http://nrn.com/consumer-trends/fine-dining-traffic-growth-outpaces-other-segents (accessed February 28, 2015). "Fast Food in the US," *EuroMonitor International*, November 1, 2014. Accessed February 28, 2015.http://www.euromonitor.com/fast-food-in-the-us/report.
2. Restaurant Opportunities Centers United (ROC United), *The Great Service Divide: Occupational Segregation & Inequality in the US Restaurant Industry.* (New York, NY: Restaurant Opportunities Centers United, 2014).

3. Ibid.
4. Part 146 of Title 12 of the Official Compilation of Codes, Rules, and Regulations of the State of New York (Cited as NYCRR 146), New York State Department of Labor, http://www.labor.ny.gov/formsdocs/wp/CR146.pdf (accessed February 27, 2015).
5. "The Capital Grille—A Darden Restaurants Brand." *The Capital Grille*, <http://www.darden.com/restaurants/capitalgrille
6. http://investor.darden.com/files/doc_financials/071814-10k_v001_x2ipxc.pdf.
7. http://investor.darden.com/files/doc_financials/071814-10k_v001_x2ipxc.pdf.
8. "Corporate Profile: Darden Restaurants Inc.," *Reuters Knowledge Direct*, LexisNexis Academic, January 5, 2015.http://www.lexisnexis.com/hottopics/lnacademic/
9. "Awards and Accolades." *Awards.* n.p., n.d., <https://www.thecapitalgrille.com/the-experience/awards>.
10. Kerri Adams, "The Capital Grille: A Fine-Dining Chain Success." *Foodabletv.com*, October 01, 2014. <http://www.foodabletv.com/blog/2014/9/29/the-capital-grille-a-fine-dining-chain-success>.
11. "Lawsuit: Capital Grille Denied Opportunities to Minority Workers." *CBS Local*, January 31, 2012. <http://chicago.cbslocal.com/2012/01/31/lawsuit-capital-grille-denied-opportunities-to-minority-workers/>.
12. Sandra Pedicini, "Almost 20,000 Join Darden Restaurants Lawsuit." *The Orlando Sentinel*, January 9, 2014. <http://articles.orlandosentinel.com/2014-01-09/business/os-darden-lawsuit-20140109_1_darden-restaurants-lawsuit-plaintiffs>.
13. Barbara Liston, "No Class-Action Suit for Darden Restaurant Staff, U.S. Judge Rules." *Reuters*, September 5, 2014. <http://www.reuters.com/article/2014/09/05/usa-florida-darden-idUSL1N0R61YG20140905>.
14. "Protestors Target Capital Grille Over Thanksgiving Plans." *Yahoo News*, <http://news.yahoo.com/video/capital-grille-employees-protest-holiday-141500115.html>.
15. "City of Pittsburgh—Meeting of City Council on 11/19/2013 at 10:00 AM." <https://pittsburgh.legistar.com/MeetingDetail.aspx?ID=275293&GUID=FE2CA538-1014-4A09-91AA-7E2025F8D77D&Search=>.

[4]

MEXICAN FOOD

Climbing the Ladder

The Mexican taco stand epitomizes the ubiquitous street-food culture of Mexico—particularly Mexico City, which has been named
one of the top ten cities for street food in the world.[1] Fifty-eight percent of Mexicans eat street food at least once a week;[2] street food
has impacted food made in the home and in the fanciest restaurants
throughout Mexico.

For her part, a street taco vendor epitomizes the notion of
moving up the ladder of Mexican life. For many American entrepreneurs, including the founder of the largest taco restaurant in
America, Taco Bell, turning the taco stand into an internationally
recognized brand represented just that. Unfortunately, the company has not represented mobility for most workers in Taco Bell or
for the millions of workers in most Mexican fast-food restaurants
in America. Instead, most Mexican fast-food restaurants provide
minimum wage jobs with no benefits and little or no mobility up
the ladder. See Table 4.1.

At least one Mexican fast-food restaurant company, Chipotle,
has decided to make internal mobility a core business practice. And
many other high-road Mexican restaurant companies manage to
provide livable wages, benefits, and internal promotion while still

Table 4.1 LOW-ROAD RESTAURANTS

	$10+ Wage for Non-Tipped Workers	Hourly Wage for Tipped Workers Exceeds Minimum	Paid Sick Days	Promotion Practices	Stars
Baja Fresh					
Del Taco		n/a*			
Moe's Southwest Grill		n/a*			
Qdoba Mexican Grill		n/a*			
Rubio's		n/a*			
Taco Bell		n/a*			
Taco Bueno					
Taco Cabana		n/a*			

*no tipped employees.

serving affordable, quick Mexican food. These restaurants, more than any others, have helped make the dream of moving up the ladder a reality for the Mexican street vendor. See Table 4.2.

TACO BELL

Glen William Bell Jr. was born in 1923 and grew up in California in the midst of the Great Depression. His family struggled to make ends meet: Bell's mother made his clothes from bleached cement sacks, and his family often found itself unable to pay rent or put food on the table.[3] As a teenager, Bell spent summers growing and harvesting potatoes, then selling them for a penny a pound.[4]

Bell served in the marines during World War II, where his primary responsibility was serving meals to his fellow soldiers.[5] After the war, his entrepreneurial and food-service experiences merged with the opening of his first restaurant, a drive-in hamburger stand called Bell's Burgers.[6] Bell's was modeled after another restaurant in San Bernadino, Mac and Dick McDonald's, which offered similar fare in a fast, made-to-order setting. Bell would soon sell this restaurant to family members, but it was the first of many fast-food restaurant ventures he'd initiate in the late 1940s and early 1950s.[7]

Observing the trajectory of McDonald's success in this period, Bell moved away from hamburgers and focused his ensuing ventures on bringing Americanized Mexican food to a fast-food setting.[8] His approach retained some basic principles of Mexican food, with some elements of authenticity sacrificed in the name of expediency: instead of using soft tortillas, he fried them—"crisp shells ready to be filled"—using a wire holder of his own design.[9] He found tacos to be a more satisfying item to sell than hamburgers because customers' orders were almost always the same and the menu items were easier to assemble.

Table 4.2 HIGH-ROAD RESTAURANTS

	$10+ Wage for Non-Tipped Workers	Hourly Wage for Tipped Workers Exceeds Minimum	Paid Sick Days	Promotion Practices	Stars
Bogota Latin Bistro *Brooklyn, NY*	💵		✓	←	★★
Café Platano Salvadoran Cuisine *Berkeley, CA*	💵	$+		←	★★
Casa Romero *Boston, MA*	💵	$+		←	★★
Chipotle *National*	💵	n/a*	✓	←	★★
Cosecha *Oakland, CA*	💵	$+		←	★★
Crema *New York, NY*	💵	$+	✓	←	★★

Restaurant	(cash)	$+	(temp)	(arrow)	(stars)
El Fuego *Philadelphia, PA*	💵	$+	●	←	★★
La Casa Del Caballo *Houston, TX*			●	←	★
La Palapa *New York, NY*	💵		●	←	★★
Los Moles *Emeryville, CA*	💵	$+	●	n/a	★★
Maya Restaurant *Los Angeles, CA*	💵	$+		n/a	★★
Racion *Los Angeles, CA*	💵	$+		←	★
Tamales La Oaxaque *Oakland, CA*	💵	$+	●	←	★★

*no tipped employees.

Bell's first taco restaurant went to his first wife following their divorce in the early 1950s.[10] He would quickly turn to other similar ventures with new partners, including restaurants called Taco Tia (for which Bell sold his shares to partner Al McDonald following disagreements over expansion models[11]) and El Taco, launched with three other partners.

Throughout these early businesses, Bell hoped to open a taco restaurant company on his own.

In 1962, he sold his shares of El Taco and started Taco Bell.[12] To grow as quickly as possible, Bell decided to sell his first franchise in 1965.[13] By 1967, there were 100 Taco Bell locations.[14] By 1977, there were 759 locations in 38 states with over 7,000 employees. Of the 759 restaurants, 430 (56 percent) were franchises.[15]

In 1978, PepsiCo. bought the company for over $130 million, with Bell receiving a share of approximately $32 million.[16] By 1987, the company's twenty-fifth anniversary, there were 2,700 Taco Bell restaurants worldwide, with sales exceeding $1.5 billion per year; by 1996, there were 6,890 restaurants with sales of $4.8 billion annually. [17]

In 1997, Yum! Brands, the restaurant division of Pepsi Co., became its own corporation, comprising Taco Bell, KFC, and Pizza Hut. Today, Taco Bell locations number more than 6,000, including more than 350 international locations in 20 countries. For its part, Yum! has become the largest restaurant corporation in the world.[18]

Taco Bell's growth has continued to rely heavily on franchising. Only about 20 percent of Taco Bell restaurants are company-owned,[19] and franchisees use Taco Bell's branding, marketing, and other intellectual property in exchange for royalties and other fees.[20] In the United States, the company plans to add 2,000 restaurants by 2022, while adding 1,300 restaurants and an additional $2 billion in system sales internationally by 2023.[21]

The State of the Food

Taco Bell makes few claims about the healthiness, freshness, or quality of its food ingredients; that might be with good reason. The company has been at the center of numerous food-safety controversies.

In 2000, up to $50 million worth of Taco Bell-branded shells were recalled by the company for containing genetically modified corn not approved for human consumption.[22] In 2011, an Alabama law firm filed a lawsuit against Taco Bell alleging false advertising after the restaurant used the terms "seasoned ground beef" and "seasoned beef" because, according to the complaint, the "meat mixture sold by Taco Bell restaurants contains binders and extenders and does not meet the minimum requirements set by the U.S. Department of Agriculture to be labeled as 'beef."[23-24] One attorney claimed that Taco Bell's meat was tested and found to contain less than 35 percent beef. Taco Bell fired back, insisting that the product is 88 percent beef, not 35 percent.[25] The Alabama law firm dropped its lawsuit after Taco Bell published the full list of ingredients.[26]

In 2006, the CDC identified the source of an E. coli outbreak in New Jersey, New York, Pennsylvania, Delaware, and South Carolina to be Taco Bell. Seventy-one people got sick. Of these, three-quarters were hospitalized, and eight "developed a type of kidney failure called hemolytic-uremic syndrome (HUS)." Public health investigators identified a few ingredients eaten more often by the ill persons than the well persons: lettuce, cheddar cheese, and ground beef—all common ingredients in many Taco Bell menu items.[27]

Again, in 2012, the Center for Disease Control (CDC) linked a ten-state outbreak of Salmonella enteritidis to Taco Bell. Although a specific food was not identified, the CDC did identify Taco Bell as the source of the widespread outbreak. As of January 19, 2012, sixty-eight individuals had reported cases of being infected with the outbreak strain of Salmonella enteritidis in ten states.[28] There were forty-three cases reported in Texas, sixteen in Oklahoma, two in Kansas, one in Iowa, one in Michigan, one in Missouri, one in Nebraska, one in New Mexico, one Ohio, and one in Tennessee.[29]

These food-safety concerns have extended to Taco Bell's international locations. In 2015, when Greg Creed, the former CEO of Taco Bell, became the new CEO of Yum!, it was thought to be "a pivotal time for its operations in China, where it gets about half of its revenue. The company has been trying to rebuild trust with customers there after one of its suppliers was investigated for selling food with too much antibiotics."[30]

Working at Taco Bell

Yum! Brands and McDonald's are two of the largest employers of low-wage workers, but have "earned strong profits throughout the postrecession recovery."[31] In 2013, Yum! Brand's CEO was paid $22 million.[32] Chris Owens of the National Employment Law Project estimates that "It would take a full-time, minimum-wage worker more than 930 years to earn as much as the chief executive officer of Yum! Brands. . . ."[33]

Until 2012, one of the most well-known labor disputes involving Taco Bell did not focus on its own employees. The Coalition of Immokalee Workers (CIW), a farmworker-organizing group in Southwestern Florida, had been fighting for over fifteen years to win better wages and working conditions for tomato pickers. For much of the fight, their arguments fell on the deaf ears of the tomato packaging plant, Pacific Tomato Growers and other farmers.[34] Farm workers around Immokalee were earning 1.3 cents per pound of tomatoes.[35] Since the 1990s the tomato business has seen nine major slavery cases brought under half the workers in the Florida fields: workers kept in chains, locked behind high fences, beaten if they refused to work, and threatened with guns.[36] It was not until CIW put pressure on consumers that things started to change. Their first target was Taco Bell. After four years of demonstrations, petitions, hunger strikes, boycotts, and shareholder votes, in 2005 "Taco Bell became the first company to sign the agreement for Fair Food." Other fast food competitors eventually followed.[37] This pressure led to the Fair Food Agreement, providing a raise of one penny per pound for the tomatoes they harvest. This would make the difference between making $50/day to $80/day.[38]

It was not until 2012 that Taco Bell's own, equally impoverished workers began to demand change publicly. Starting in 2012, Taco Bell has been at the center of fast food workers' strikes across the country and across the globe.[39] *New York Times* reporter Steven Greenhouse reported on one of the strikes. "Late Wednesday morning, one hundred people protested in front of a Taco Bell on Eight Mile Road in Detroit, with organizers saying that eleven of the restaurant's employees were on strike. One Taco Bell worker, Sharise Stitt, 27, joined the strike, saying the $8.09 she earns after five years there was insufficient to support her family ... After taxes, she has about $900 a month to feed and clothe her three children. They receive food stamps."[40] According to NELP, the estimated annual cost of taxpayer-subsidized public assistance to Yum! Brands' employees (Taco Bell, Pizza Hut, and KFC) is $648 million.[41] Meanwhile, Yum! Brands is in great financial condition: in 2012, the CEO was compensated $14.1 million with company profits estimated at $1.59 billion.[42]

Taco Bell has also been at the center of numerous lawsuits over employee rights. From 2003 to 2013, 28,000 Taco Bell workers filed a class action lawsuit in California claiming that they were not given proper breaks in accordance with California state law. The judge ruled that the company was not liable for the practices of its franchise operators.[43] In 2013, the National Labor Relations Board ruled that corporate chains are liable for the labor law violations of their franchise operators. Nevertheless, most lawsuits against Taco Bell restaurants have focused on franchise operators. One of the most egregious cases emerged in 2000, when a franchisee owner of 24 Taco Bell restaurants in Massachusetts and Rhode Island was found to be in violation of federal child labor regulations and agreed to pay $44,850 in fines. The owner had employed sixty-nine children in violation of the FLSA's child labor provisions between 1997–1999. All the minors, who were between 14 and 15 years old, were found working as late as 11 P.M. and for more than three hours on school days.[44]

Anthony's Story: Dismantling the Myth of Mobility

Anthony Peeples's description of his hometown LaPort, Indiana, is bleak, almost dystopian: "It's the typical postindustrial town. All that's left are abandoned factories, and the three to four factories that are still around. All we have to work at are those three, or Walmart, or the chain restaurants."

Peeples grew up in working-class poverty. "My mom worked at McDonald's, the YMCA, and for a group that helped the developmentally disabled. My Dad worked food service in the state prison. We lived in my Grandma's house when she moved in with her new husband. But my folks couldn't afford the bills. I remember a couple of occasions where we'd get rooms at a local hotel because my folks couldn't afford to pay the electricity and water bills and they got shut off, in the middle of January."

Anthony's parents worked hard to send him to Catholic school in the suburbs. "There's a huge wealth gap. Outside of town there's a bunch of rich people. My parents sent me to Catholic school out there, and I'd have rattier clothes than the other kids. It was the only Catholic school in town, and it was a horrible experience. My brother was miserable going there. We finally went to public school after we couldn't afford it anymore." Even in public school, though, Anthony remembers "just not having everything that the other kids had."

In high school, Anthony found himself in a group of friends who felt fairly isolated from the rest of society due to their environment and circumstances. "A lot of my friends developed drug habits; a lot of my graduating class died of heroin overdose. All of the stress of society weighed on them—and they found an outlet. Either they became a cog in the machine, working at one of the chains or the factories, or they developed crippling drug addiction, or they became criminals. A lot of my friends got into dealing or selling drugs, or selling stolen items. LaPort is ranked number 9 out of 100 on crime index. All my old friends from high school are the rough individuals."

Running for the Border?
Anthony started working at Taco Bell while still in high school, out of necessity. "My parents were not doing great. I needed the extra cash to get a car, but a good percentage of what I earned I gave them to help out with the bills and rent. It was about half of what I made."

Anthony was lured to Taco Bell by their supposedly higher pay than McDonald's. "They paid $6.25 an hour. During the interview, the manager told me 'This is why we pay you better than McDonald's. We are better. I expect my employees to go the extra mile."

"I was supposed to work the line, but they expected so much out of their employees. They expected me to come in and work for so many hours; and everything I did wasn't good enough. I was responsible for doing the cash register, doing the drive-through window, being on the food line, enough wasn't enough at any point. It was a horrible experience."

"During the day, I'd be the only cook on the line. On the third or fourth day, I was completely overworked, and the manager was being an asshole. He was so condescending to me. He'd say, 'You're too slow, what's wrong with you? Move faster."

"I would come in for the morning shift at 10 A.M. I'd work the fryer with no training. There's no good training for these positions, they just throw you into the fire. The manager would be sitting there, saying 'We've got raw chips, you're an a**hole, what's wrong with you? Get out here, do this.' They kept moving me around. It was degrading, and they didn't pay well enough, as they said. I'd work the bathrooms, I'd be pushed around in a new position every week. When they'd say, 'What's wrong with you, why can't you do this?' I'd think 'You're telling me to do new things that I didn't learn before. You didn't give me any proper training.'"

Anthony can recall several times that the manager almost fired him. "One time they almost fired me because my ID badge fell into the fryer. They had to empty the frying oil." Anthony reports that no one was trained to use the fryer, full of boiling oil. "Everybody gets hurt. Grease pops out of the fryer and gets onto any exposed skin. It hurts. It also ruins your complexion—you get all kinds of zits from standing over hot oil all day."

Despite the lack of training and the difficult and dangerous work environment, there was no talk of benefits for sick or injured workers, like workers' compensation or a sick day. "We all worked when we were sick."

Worst of all, for the supposedly higher pay, management expected and encouraged workers to rat on one another. "One of my co-workers quit shortly before I did. She was in tears about how badly they treated everybody. She was telling me—and started crying—about all the stuff she heard others talking to management about me and her."

Anthony observed an incredibly high turnover rate; the only workers who stayed were those who talked to management about their co-workers. "The company encourages and conditions people to rat on other employees. They make it seem like they pay you so well—like a dollar or fifty cents above the minimum wage. They said, 'We'll treat you well, so take care of us.' It was not really good pay—we were expected to do a lot of work. Despite what they tell you, it's not good pay."

Anthony also noticed that the myth of Taco Bell workers being all teenagers like himself was also not true. "Of the 20 [people] that worked there, there were only a few teenagers like me. There were mostly adults working there. Some had kids. Most only stayed a few months. The company tried to make it seem like you could live off $6.25, and that you might even make it to $7. But most people left because the pay was so bad. It was a revolving door."

There was not real mobility that Anthony saw at the Taco Bell. "There were just the entry level workers and the manager, Vernon. It was the dictatorship of Vernon. Some of the employees who ratted on each other got fifty cents more. But we were all doing the same work. There was no real ladder. They didn't offer any opportunities to move up that were legitimate."

Even Vernon, the manager, did not earn much more than the line-level workers. "Vernon had worked there over twenty years, and he's still there now. He would always complain about his pay. He'd always complain 'The workers are paid so well they get more than me.'"

Like so many of his coworkers, Anthony eventually left to find a better-paying job in pizza delivery. "Everyone [at Taco Bell] understood that the myth of being paid more wasn't true."

Many of Peeples's coworkers from Taco Bell still work there. "We don't have much to compare it to. I grew up and still live in a city that's overpopulated by Walmart, McDonald's, Taco Bell, Arby's, every chain there is. That's pretty much all you have to work with." Accordingly, the standards for what constitutes a better job are fairly low. "I left because mom and pop restaurants might not pay that much better, but at least I don't get treated like an animal. I would have taken a pay cut to work somewhere where I was treated like a human being."

By the time he graduated from high school, Anthony hoped to escape the same fate of many of his classmates and coworkers by learning to be a union carpenter. "My uncle was a carpenter, and I always looked up to my uncle. I had always done things with my hands—welding, working in factories, cooking, bartending. I took building trades in high school and really enjoy it. The high school would buy a site, and we spent two semesters building a house." Unfortunately, Anthony's high school dream was not to be. "I graduated in 2008, at the height of the economic crisis. It was also the height of the housing crisis. All my dreams of being a carpenter completely washed away. I was stuck delivering pizzas. I began to see—the same thing my folks went through, I'm stuck in the same thing."

THE HIGH ROAD: CHIPOTLE

Monty Moran grew up in Boulder, Colorado, in a progressive household in which his parents—his father a biology professor and his mother was a psychologist, social worker, and artist–welcomed other, more disadvantaged families to live with them. "My parents were very open to everything and everyone. I grew up with very diverse people coming in and out of our home, and watching my parents being very welcoming of everybody." At age 15, Moran got a job as a line cook at a Dairy Queen in Boulder, where he learned more than just cooking: "There was a mental hospital across the street, and a lot of mentally ill and homeless people would come into the restaurant. These people would come in and sit and wrap themselves around a coffee for more than an hour. Their nutrition would come from the cream on the coffee."

"Every now and then I'd have a rejected burger from another customer, and I'd take it to them to eat. I'd spend an hour or more talking to them, during times when the restaurant was slow. I got to know so many people who had so many difficult and diverse backgrounds. They came from all walks of life, and I'd get to learn about their backgrounds. I was fascinated."

As often happens in states that have a lower minimum wage, the Dairy Queen bent the rules by paying Moran—a kitchen worker who did *not* receive tips—the Colorado minimum wage for tipped workers, $2.35 an hour. "But still, I loved working there. I loved my job. I learned so much about people's backgrounds, people's plights, people's personal dramas. Some of it was mental illness, some of it was a mental block. They were not made to believe they were worth anything or that they could be successful. There were psychological obstacles that had been put there by their parents, by people who had beaten them or molested them. I tried to help them overcome that. I loved them. I valued them."

After college, Moran moved to California and took a series of jobs in the insurance industry. His first job was claims adjuster for a big insurance company—"an extraordinarily corrupt business. I got to see the difference between honest and dishonest people"— and later, after going to law school, as an attorney defending against insurance claims.

"At first, they wanted me to defend big corporations in products liability cases. I felt like a trained monkey in a suit, and I didn't like it. I told the firm to let me get involved with actual trials—something no one else wanted to do." Moran got his wish, and took assignments defending companies against fraudulent insurance claims. "It'd be a few lawyers who would set up and stage accidents, get a doctor to sign off on some ginnied up medical bills. I'd have to break it open. I did hundreds of cases like that. I'd have fifty-five open cases at one time. I'd get good at knowing when people are telling the truth, and when they were lying. I've become a really good poker player—I know when people are lying. I could catch them in a lie, then I'd get the case dismissed."

After getting married, Moran moved back to Colorado in 1996 and began work as a trial lawyer working at a large firm in Denver. Moran is careful to point out that he worked *at* the firm, not necessarily for it. "The founder of that law firm told me, 'To be a great lawyer, a great leader, you have to develop your own practice, your own clients.' I said okay, I don't know how to do that—but what a challenge!" Moran approached the challenge of building clients in a new city by immersing himself in the work. "I treated the smallest case as if they were big deals. Every client who came to me, I took their problems more seriously than they did. It was very stressful, but the clients walked away from their first meeting with me feeling, 'Okay, someone's going to help me.' I was hell-bent for leather on solving their problem. I was good at it, but I worked really hard because I was insecure that I wasn't good. I'd be billing $100 an hour, which I now know is nothing for a lawyer, I developed a reputation among people who said, 'Go to that guy, he'll care about it.' The business was flooding in."

However, what at first gave Moran an ego boost later turned into a challenge. "I'd take on more and more clients, and I got busier and busier and busier. I felt great, I had lots of clients, I was billing more hours than anyone in the law firm. My ego said, 'this is good.' It was all, 'me, me, me'; I wanted to be the one to do all the work. As I got even busier, that became my Achilles heel. I couldn't do more—but I kept saying yes."

The necessary expansion of Moran's legal practice included hiring newer, younger attorneys, then handing clients off. In order to make the client reassignments work, it required a deft managerial touch from Moran, one that ensured the culture of the practice was adhered to by his staff. "I told the junior attorneys: 'Here's what we're going to be like. We're going to solve people's problems.' I realized I needed the right type of people—I had to hire carefully. I made mistakes, but I had to hire people who could love that vision and were completely committed to that vision."

"The lawyers I hired were excellent, but I needed to create a culture in which they could learn and be at their best very quickly. Most law firms are reluctant to give young lawyers client contact, for fear they'll steal the clients and go start their own firm. I realized I wanted to create an environment where people wanted to stay."

Moran uses a parenting analogy: "It's like, if you love your kids, and let them be free, they'll come back at Christmas. But if you stifle them and keep them weak, they'll never come back. You have to empower people, to allow them to be at their best. Give them the latitude to leave you, and create an environment that pays them well and treats them well."

With a supportive, positive culture, Moran's practice flourished, and his stable of clients grew in size and profile. One of those clients was Chipotle, a small restaurant company that Moran's high school and college friend Steve Ells had founded in 1993. Ells, a culinary academy graduate, sold San Francisco-style burritos at Chipotle as a means of generating the income he needed to open his dream fine dining establishment. When Chipotle took off—with a significant investment from McDonald's in 1998—Ells decided to focus his energy there. Now he wanted Moran to join him and bring his workplace culture to a new scale and industry.

Ells' courtship of Moran persisted for five years. "I had been at the firm for ten years," Moran recalls. "It was wonderful. The firm was growing quickly. The lawyers loved being there. Steve said, 'Do you think you can do this at Chipotle?' I said, 'No, I'm a lawyer.' Steve said, 'What you really are is a natural-born leader.' I thought about it and thought about it, and after a series of fits and starts I said yes."

Bringing the Culture to Chipotle

Although he later became co-CEO with Steve Ells, Moran started as general counsel in 2009, when the company had ten thousand employees. McDonalds had 92 percent ownership, and the company was about to go public. "I agreed to join Chipotle because by the time I started, the writing was on the wall that McDonald's was going to part ways with the company. I didn't want to work for McDonald's. I wanted to create an environment [at Chipotle] that was vibrant, alive, smart, competitive, fun, opportunistic, optimistic, excited, exciting, smart, challenging. I hired people who challenged me, and challenged each other. I wanted people to make each other better."

In 2006, McDonald's divested all of its stock in Chipotle. "They decided to focus on what they do best: burgers and fries." Moran set out to assess the employee culture at Chipotle and how it could be modified moving forward. As a counterpoint to traditional American fast-food culture and as one of the first major chains to make claims about the quality of its ingredient sourcing, Chipotle had a cultural advantage over its competition. "Chipotle had a relatively optimistic culture because it was a cool brand and the food was good. People were proud to work at Chipotle as opposed to traditional fast-food restaurants. Chipotle had this 'food with integrity' philosophy. Steve and the purchasing department started to get better quality ingredients. They were focused on sustainability, healthfulness, preservation of the family farm, land stewardship, and animal husbandry. For all those reasons, the employees were excited." Still, problems remained visible: upward mobility among employees was no better than among competitors, which was evident in the racial stratification of the employees. As Moran recalls, "the crew [line staff] was 87 percent Hispanic. The management was a lot more white."

Before *Undercover Boss* became a show on CBS, Moran used its premise to gather insight on his company. "I went to train for 10 weeks in one of the restaurants. We set it up so that I was a manager-in-training, and only the store manager knew that I was the president and new co-CEO. The way the system worked back then, the company would hire managers-in-training from the outside—mostly white people with some background in fast food. They'd bring them into Chipotle, train them on the grill, on the prep line, the front line. They'd tell them 'here's how you do the books,'etc." In his ten weeks as a manager-in-training, Moran came away more impressed by the Chipotle crew, which was mostly Latino, than his mostly white fellow management trainees. "The crew knew the food better than anyone. But the other managers-in-training with me at that store, who had come from other fast-food restaurants, were super unimpressive. They were not hospitable, not caring for the crew. I said, 'Why are we hiring these people?' They were brought in for their fast-food management experience, as if that was something good."

For their part, the employees who were training Moran to be manager seemed complacent with their employment level. "I'd ask them, 'What do you want to do in 3–5 years? What more do you want in life?' They'd say, 'This is great. I love it.' We had the right people. But they didn't have cause to believe that they could want

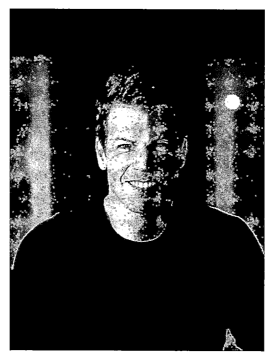

Monty Moran.

more and realistically get it. If I asked them, 'Do you want to be a manager?' they'd give me a funny look as if to say, 'What's the catch?' It was as if I was asking them, 'Do you want to win the lottery?' The answer was, 'Sure, I'd love to, but how would that ever happen?'"

Moran's immersion in a Chipotle restaurant led to a radicalized approach to management structure, one that he announced unilaterally to a group of store general managers shortly thereafter: within two years, all incoming Chipotle general managers would be promoted from within. The reaction? "Their jaws hit the floor. In the past there were occasionally people who had moved through the ranks—like 20 percent of managers had come from the line. But I wanted to turn that on its head."

Ells embraced Moran's concept—"He said, 'Cool, how do we do it?'" as Moran recalls—and the two set out to institute changes at the store level. "We wanted to recognize managers who did the job in an enlightened way," Moran says.

In the new managerial model, Chipotle recognized that the general manager of a given restaurant is the most important cog in creating a culture of promotion and empowerment. Rather than promoting exceptional general managers to roles that separated them from customers and line-level employees, Chipotle created a new "restaurateur" designation that recognized managerial excellence while still leaving a connection to restaurant culture. "A restaurateur is a general manager who builds a culture of all top performers [among their line-level staff] who are empowered to achieve a high standard. I wanted to go out and find all the general managers in the company who empowered others to achieve high standards."

Ells and Moran went to the extreme measure of traveling to every Chipotle location to interview every general manager working for the company. "People said, 'That's crazy.' I said, 'Well, we'll just do it.' We started bringing them to the office to do the interviews, and then we realized we needed to go to them. So we flew to every restaurant, interviewed the crew to find out whether general managers were producing all top performers with a good culture that was thriving and running well as a result. For those that didn't make the cut, we'd talk to them about how to do better, and for the most part, people were willing to sit and listen and find out how."

After hundreds of visits and several years defining the program, Moran and his team have developed a very specific career ladder, with very clear and specific benchmarks for workers to move along a much more graduated path. All workers in the entire company receive biannual performance reviews, and the requirements for moving up the ladder are posted in the back of each store. "If you are clear about what to do, people do it."

General managers are now recognized, above all else, for moving everyone along this ladder. "We measure the managers based on whether they are enlightened—whether they create a culture of empowerment and aren't just going around yelling at people, and whether they develop other people along the way." Moran defines empowerment as "feeling confident in your ability and encouraged by your circumstances such that you feel motivated and at liberty to advance—meaning that you know that the person you work for cares for you, believes in you, challenges you, pushes you, wants the best for you. The foundational principle is that each of us is rewarded based on our effectiveness in making the people around us better."

Chipotle's imperatives of empowerment are evident throughout its business practices. Workers are involved in the interviewing process for new applicants, and each is asked to look for the thirteen characteristics of a good team member that Moran has developed: conscientious, respectful, hospitable, high energy, infectiously enthusiastic, happy, presentable, smart, polite, motivated, ambitious, curious, and honest.

Moran's desire to continue to improve as an employer appears genuine: Chipotle pays at least $1 higher than most other fast food restaurants, and Moran is now considering a $10 starting wage in higher cost-of-living markets. During his interview for this book, he asked for a list of policies Chipotle could consider that would improve the lives of their workers. He followed up during the weeks that followed, asking for data on the cost-impacts of policies like paid sick days and paid vacation time, which I provided. A few months later, in June 2015, Chipotle announced that it was providing paid sick days, paid vacation time, and tuition reimbursements to all its several hundred thousand employees nationwide. So while the company still has a way to go to provide livable starting wages,

Chipotle is now providing much higher than average benefits and mobility opportunities, very unique in the industry.

"We hire great people; we think they deserve it. We're looking for people without any regard to experience or education. The thirteen characteristics we're looking for have almost nothing to do with socioeconomic background or education; it's about whether you were raised well and have a good human spirit. Once we get those people, they become managers, fast."

Chipotle's higher pay and employee development program have paid off in lower-than-average turnover. Still, "It's higher than we'd like it to be," and something Moran says the company is working to improve.

Moran also acknowledges that Chipotle is not immune from making mistakes, which is evident in the fact that the company has been sued for wage and hour violations. "Class action lawsuits don't get my attention because I'm a lawyer and I know that, in those lawsuits, the lawyer's making way more money than the workers. But workers report problems, legal violations all the time—and they know I won't stand for it." Moran distributes his personal number to line-level workers at stores he visits. "They never abuse the privilege. They email or call me and tell me, 'Hey this manager is abusive,' or 'that someone is being harassed,' and we take it really seriously. We have anonymous hotlines for people to call if they fear reprisal—I don't want anyone fearing reprisal in this company. That's not the kind of company I'm trying to build."

Told of the National Restaurant Association's argument that higher wages and a professionalized career ladder is not necessary because most fast-food restaurant workers are teenagers or young people earning extra cash on the side, Moran responds, "That's hogwash. That's not who these workers are. To work at Chipotle requires skill and love.

"People are important. People are the only things that matter. Plus, people who care are more productive, less sick, more loyal, turn over less frequently."

Case Study: Pedro

Pedro was born in San Miguel de Allende, Guanajato, Mexico, to a comfortable, working-class family. His father was a contractor; his mother stayed home to care for Pedro and his two sisters. In the early 1990s, when Pedro was 8 years old, he and his family were forced to emigrate to the United States in the midst of an economic downturn in Mexico. "The devaluation of the peso was terrible. My dad had outstanding loans with his company, and found himself in a very tough situation financially. So he found himself making a very tough decision, which was to migrate to the United States."

Pedro's family travelled first to San Miguel, in northern Mexico, then entered the United States on six-month visitor visas. "My dad's plan was not to come and visit; his plan was to stay."

The family went first to Chicago, where Pedro's mother had a family member and a potential construction job for Pedro's father. When that work never materialized, the family moved to Denver, where Pedro's uncle had been living and working for eight years. Even with this connection, the learning curve was steep. "You can imagine, as an 8-year-old boy, the culture shock, going to the United States, not speaking the language. There was hardly anyone speaking Spanish in the school. Some teachers had aides who were bilingual, but very few. I got pretty good at English within three or four months because I had no choice."

Pedro's parents found their first jobs in restaurants. "I remember they were working at Vietnamese restaurants, both mom and dad. My dad was the dishwasher for the morning and night, and my mom would be the helper at night. They were not home much for first part of our lives in Denver." Pedro's sister, three years older, took care of Pedro and his other sister.

After spending a year in Pedro's uncle's apartment, the family moved into their own one-bedroom apartment in the same complex, using the uncle's social security number to bypass immigration complications. "At night, we'd pull out inflatable mattresses and put those in the living room and sleep there. We lived there for a couple of years, and eventually moved out of that apartment complex and into a two-bedroom."

Pedro's parents took second jobs to finance the move to a larger apartment. After the parents washed dishes Monday through Friday, the entire family would spend the weekend cleaning a large conference and banquet restaurant in downtown Denver. "We'd go there early, like 5 in the morning, Saturdays and Sundays. My mom and dad would take us to help them because the two of them couldn't get it done on time. We'd vacuum, clean mats, sweep floors, take out the trash, do dishes left from night before. It was fun as a kid to do that. It was an opportunity to go and do something. It was a big part of developing my work ethic— to value menial labor, understand it, work hard. I saw my parents do it, they would teach us those things. That shaped me into the kind of person I am now. I had experience in restaurants at a very early age."

Entering the Restaurant Industry

Pedro got his own job when he turned 14. "My mom's uncle had opened a Mexican restaurant. You can't work at that age, legally, but my parents wanted me to continue to learn, and they asked my uncle to give me a job sweeping the parking lot, picking up dishes, filling up waters, cleaning the bathroom, being the busboy."

Once he was of age to work legally, Pedro looked for a job that paid better, and one that would employ him without looking into his immigration status. At 17 he was hired to work a stock position at a Walgreens. He earned multiple promotions from there while also graduating from high school early. Through it all, his focus was, by necessity, on making money. "I became passionate about having my own money, earning my own money. I knew my situation—I knew I wasn't 'legal' at the time. I knew that to be able to apply for any type of financial aid to go to college, it was going to be hard because I was not documented. So my only option was to work. I really focused on that."

The focus paid off, and after five years—after stints in stock, checkout, photo department, pharmacy, and as an assistant manager—Pedro was promoted to general manager of his Walgreens store. "I had built a nice lifestyle. I had a car and an apartment." Pedro was saving money and was sharing portions of his salary with his parents.

When Walgreens discovered that Pedro was an undocumented worker, he was dismissed. He sold his car and began looking for work where he knew he could get it—restaurants. "It's a lot easier to find a job that way when your documents are not in order. There's always a job in the restaurant industry."

Pedro's first jobs after Walgreens were server jobs paying $2.50 an hour, the Colorado minimum wage for tipped workers at the time. His income fluctuated wildly. "As a server, sometimes I would have money to pay the bills, and sometimes not. I lived with a couple of guys from Peru and Costa Rica, sharing a two-bedroom apartment. They were also in the restaurant industry. We had to have each other's backs. Sometimes one of us had to pay rent, and the others had to pay us back later."

Working at Chipotle

Pedro was referred to one of Chipotle's original Denver locations by a friend who promised him, "There are opportunies to advance." Pedro started as a prep cook in 2005 earning Chipotle's entry wage, which was then "$7.50 or $8.00"—well above the minimum wage. The work was invigorating: "I immediately fell in love with it. It was really hard physically. I'd get blisters from cutting, because I'd never cooked before. But I fell in love with the cooking,"

Pedro skyrocketed through the store ranks at Chipotle—from crew to kitchen manager, then, after a few months, to service manager. Months later he was assistant manager, which is also referred to as "apprentice general manager." With each promotion came an hourly raise between $1.00 and $1.50, and beginning at assistant manager he was salaried with benefits. Within a year and a half, when his manager was called away to open a new store in Florida, Pedro was named the store's general manager. "By that time," Pedro recalls, "the restaurateur program had started, and I was really close to making [that] happen."

Having started at Chipotle before Moran's arrival and ensuing changes to the Chipotle management structure, Pedro has been witness to the developing culture of the business. From the start, "It was the people, more than anything else. It was the values and vision that the company had. It was what my dad was trying to create for us when we came from Mexico. If you work hard, you can be leaders, managers, succeed, grow with this company. The manager will notice your efforts, your desire to grow, you'll become successful. It really completely felt like what the real American dream is all about."

"What Monty brought was far beyond anybody's expectations of what this company could truly be, of truly driving people. He helped us understand what we were focusing on more than the burritos—it's a people business. He helped make it clear that this company is going to be successful only if we truly build a vision around a people culture. What Monty brought with the restaurateur program was really what it needed. The company skyrocketed after that."

When prompted to compare his managerial experiences at Walgreens and Chipotle, Pedro concedes, "I was lucky that I was given opportunities at Walgreen's; most of the time, they'd prefer to have someone who brought a ton of experience to run their stores." His ascent at Chipotle felt more organic and fluid. "It's really about your ability to make the people around you better, to develop your replacement. At Chipotle, when I moved from kitchen manger to service manager, I had to develop the kitchen manager to replace me. I had to develop someone to replace me who was as good or better than me every step of the way. That's the expectation, culture, and vision—you have to make the people around you better. You can't leave until you develop your replacement, and you're given the training tools to do that. We're a lot better than we were ten years ago—we have better tools now. But there were always tools to learn how to develop your replacement."

Pedro was promoted into Moran's new restaurateur program. As with most things at Chipotle, the program has evolved over time. "Back then, the way it worked was that the field leader would say, 'I think you're ready. You've built a great people culture, and that's reflected in the food quality, the customer service, the customer experience.' Then he had his boss, the operations director, validate it. Today, you get to become a restaurateur when you create an amazing people culture with top performers achieving high standards—when you are developing future general managers for the company."

Pedro's interview with Ells and Moran sufficiently impressed the two executives to the point that they made Pedro's Chipotle a test kitchen for new products—"where all new equipment and new recipes would be tested."

Promotion to restaurateur comes with a title as well as increased compensation, a company vehicle, and financial shares in the company. In a manner that's highly unique in the restaurant industry, increases in compensation for Chipotle employees are based not only on individual performance, but on employees' ability to develop others. According to Pedro, "You get 'people development' bonuses when you can move people from crew to general manager. If you develop a couple of general managers in one year, you can add 40–50 percent to your salary, just on people development alone."

Promotion beyond restaurateur at Chipotle is incremental, and requires gradual mentoring of additional general managers in pursuit of restaurateur status. Titles above that range from apprentice team leader to executive team director, which can come with a purview of hundreds of restaurants. All are clearly defined rungs in the Chipotle corporate ladder and are displayed at the back of stores.

Pedro recounts that every move up for him included pay increases, bonuses, and more shares in the company. Approaching his tenth year anniversary with the company, and now age 33, Pedro is one of eight executive team leaders who oversee the eight regions of Chipotle restaurants. Moran estimates that with shares, executive team leaders can earn several hundred thousand dollars annually.

Pedro continually turns conversation about Chipotle to the importance of mutual empowerment. "One of the things that we encourage people about—all the way down to the crew—we encourage them to understand our vision. In order to be successful at Chipotle, the number one thing is to elevate people around you to be as good or better than you.

"We need leaders that come from crew, because they understand our culture, our vision. What Monty always says is that you will be rewarded based on your ability to make people around you better. I just want to focus on that, continuing to develop my team leaders to be the best, and if that means I get a promotion because I've developed my replacement, then that's awesome."

NOTES

1. Andrew Bender, "The World's Top 10 Cities for Street Food," *Forbes Magazine*, September 19, 2012. Accessed January 23, 2013 <http://www.forbes.com/sites/andrewbender/2012/09/19/the-worlds-top-10-cities-for-street-food/>
2. "McCann Worldgroup Unveils "Truth About Street" Discoveries: A study of street food habits of 12,000 consumers in 25 cities in 18 Latin American countries serves up a $127 billion a year missed opportunity for brands," *McCann Worldgroup, Sao Paulo*, July 31, 2012. http://www.prnewswire.com/news-releases/mccann-worldgroup-unveils-truth-about-street-discoveries-164468896.html.
3. Debra Lee Baldwin, *Taco Titan: The Glen Bell Story* (Arlington, TX: Summit Pub. Group, 1999), 8–9.
4. Baldwin, \17.
5. Baldwin, 43.
6. Baldwin, 50-53.
7. Baldwin, 57.
8. Baldwin,. 60-63.
9. Baldwin, 64.
10. Baldwin, 66.
11. Baldwin, 71-89.
12. Baldwin, 97-101.
13. Baldwin, 107.
14. Baldwin, 132.
15. Baldwin, 182
16. Baldwin, 188.
17. Baldwin, 241.
18. Taco Bell Company Profile. Zoom Company Information, December 20, 2014. LexisNexis Academic. <http://www.lexisnexis.com/hottopics/lnacademic/>
19. Taco Bell Company Profile. Hoover's Company Records, (December 30, 2014): LexisNexis Academic. Web.
20. Ibid.

21. Taco Bell. "Taco Bell Appoints New Leadership Positions For Domestic And International Growth." December 4, 2014, <https://www.tacobell.com/Company/newsreleases/new-leadership-positions-for-domestic-and-international-growth-2014> (accessed August 17, 2015).

22. Melinda Fulmer, "Taco Bell Recalls Shells That Used Bioengineered Corn." *Los Angeles Times*, September 23, 2000. http://articles.latimes.com/2000/sep/23/news/mn-25314.

23. "Alabama Law Firm Sues Taco Bell, Claims There's Not Enough Meat in its Advertised 'Beef.'" *Inside Counsel*, January 25, 2011. <http://www.inside-counsel.com/2011/01/25/alabama-law-firm-sues-taco-bell-claims-theres-not-enough-meat-in-its-advertised-beef>

24. "Alabama Law Firm Sues Taco Bell"

25. Eliza Barclay,. "With Lawsuit Over, Taco Bell's Mystery Meat is a Mystery No Longer." *NPR*, April 19, 2011.

26. http://www.tacobell.com/Company/newsreleases/Voluntary_Lawsuit_Withdrawal_1011.

27. "Multistate Outbreak of E. coli O157 Infections, November-December 2006." E. coli, Foodborne and Diarrheal Diseases Branch, Centers for Disease Control, December 14, 2006. < http://www.cdc.gov/ecoli/2006/december/121406.htm>.

28. "Investigation Announcement: Multistate Outbreak of *Salmonella* Enteritidis Infections Linked to Restaurant Chain A." *Salmonella*, Centers for Disease Control and Prevention, Jan. 19, 2012; Alan J. Liddle, "Government Ties Taco Bell to Outbreak Investigation." *Nation's Restaurant News*, Feb. 3, 2012. < http://nrn.com/archive/government-ties-taco-bell-outbreak-investigation>.

29. Samantha Bonar,. "Taco Bell Implicated in 10-State Salmonella Outbreak." *LA Weekly*, Feb. 3, 2012.

30. Leslie Patton,. "Yum Names Niccolas Taco Bell's CEO After Creed Is Promoted." *Bloomberg*, May 21, 2014. <http://www.bloomberg.com/news/articles/2014-05-20/yum-names-niccol-as-taco-bell-s-ceo-after-creed-gets-promotion>.

31. Stephanie West, "Fast-Food Workers Face No Chance of Advancement," *Labor Press*, July 29, 2013. < http://laborpress.org/sectors/union-retail/2644-fast-food-workers-face-no-chance-of-advancement>; Data Brief, "Going Nowhere Fast: Limited Occupational Mobility in the Fast Food Industry." *National Employment Law Project*, July 2013. http://nelp.3cdn.net/84a67b124db45841d4_o0m6bq42h.pdf.

32. Allison Aubrey,. "Fast-Food CEO's Earn Supersize Salaries; Workers Earn Small Potatoes." *NPR*, April 22, 2014.

33. Christine Owens, "Trying to Raise a Family on a Fast-Food Salary." *Reuters*, Aug. 29, 2013.<http://blogs.reuters.com/great-debate/2013/08/28/trying-to-raise-a-family-on-a-fast-food-salary/>

34. Barry Estabrook,. "Building a Better Tomato." *Gastronomica: The Journal of Food and Culture* 11 no. 3, 2011: 21.

35. Daniel Zwerdling, "Farm Workers Aim to Enforce Taco Bell Deal." *NPR*, June 17, 2005. http://www.npr.org/templates/story/story.php?storyId=4708129.
36. Estabrook, 21-22.
37. Estabrook, 22.
38. Estabrook, 21.
39. NY Workers Rising, About NY Workers Rising, 2014. <www.nyworkersrising.org>
40. Steven Greenhouse, "A Day's Strike Seeks to Raise Fast-Food Pay." *The New York Times.* July 31, 2013. <http://www.nytimes.com/2013/08/01/business/strike-for-day-seeks-to-raise-fast-food-pay.html>
41. Data Brief, "Super-Sizing Public Costs: How Low Wages at Top Fast-Food Chains Leave Taxpayers Footing the Bill." *National Employment Law Project*, October 2013.. 2.
42. Ibid., 3.
43. Aaron Vehling,. "Taco Bell Workers Didn't Prove Illegal Break Policy: Judge." *Law360*, September 2, 2014.
44. News Release, "Taco Bell Franchise Chain Agrees to Pay $44,850 in Fines for Federal Child Labor Violations." *Department of Labor*, January 10, 2000. <http://www.dol.gov/whd/media/press/bowh0006.htm>.

[5]

BURGERS, BILLS, AND
NO BENEFITS

Nothing about the history of the hamburger lends any merit to its contemporary connotations of being inherently lowbrow or low quality. Some trace the origins of the hamburger to Ancient Rome, when a unique preparation of beef developed that included mixing the beef with peppercorns and wine.[1] Various minced meat precursors can be traced back to Genghis Khan and the Mongolians. In Europe, minced meat was a delicacy reserved for the upper classes.[2]

In the nineteenth century, European ships embarking on transatlantic voyages made the port of Hamburg, Germany, the central point of departure for emigrants and exports headed to America.[3] In the New World, restaurants started selling a "Hamburg steak" as an appeal to immigrants missing their homeland. The earliest recorded Hamburg steak on a restaurant menu was at Delmonico's, the original fine dining restaurant in New York City.[4] Delmonico's was the epitome of high-class food service. Even the idea of a steak in a sandwich came from aristocracy—when the English Earl of Sandwich wanted his meals served between slices of bread so as not to soil his hands while playing cards.[5]

In America, there is great controversy over who developed the exact notion of a hamburger that we see today, with the creation stories ranging from street vendors at a county fair to local restaurant owners in small town America—and in Hamburg, Germany.[6] Some of these stories include notions of concepts of beef sandwiches that people could eat while walking around a fair or going to work, but none include notions of low quality or skill.[7]

Since the arrival of the ubiquitous McDonald's restaurant chain, Americans have come to equate hamburgers with the "McJob": low-wage, seemingly low-skill, monotonous jobs reserved for entry-level or unskilled members of the workforce. Hamburgers have also become the ultimate symbol of fast food—low-quality, unhealthy items relegated to the growing portion of America that has neither the resources nor the time to eat well. And for most, low wages and lack of benefits such as earned sick leave seem to follow as a necessary part of that consumer equation.

A 2014 *New York Times* article shone a light on how the Americanized hamburger—particularly the McDonald's treatment of it—is a distinctly American condition. The article profiled fast-food employment in Denmark, where workers earn $20 an hour, as opposed to the wage of $8.90 paid by McDonald's in the United States—and the Big Mac is $5.60, as opposed to $4.80 in the United States. McDonald's workers in Denmark also receive five weeks paid vacation, paid maternity and paternity leave, and a pension plan. Employee turnover, not surprisingly, is much lower—more than 70 percent of Danish employees stay for more than a year, whereas McDonald's reports that its workers' average tenure was less than eight months.[8]

What was most remarkable about the *New York Times* piece was that the Danish burger could cost just $.80 more while workers were receiving almost two and a half times the wage plus benefits. The head of Denmark's restaurant operations at the central airport was quoted as saying "We have to acknowledge it's more expensive to operate.

But we can still make money out of it—and McDonald's does, too. Otherwise, it wouldn't be in Denmark. The company doesn't get as much profit, but the profit is shared a little differently. We don't want there to be a big difference between the richest and poorest, because poor people would just get really poor. We don't want people living on the streets. If that happens, we consider that we as a society have failed."[9]

So is the McDonald's and fast-food model in the United States the model of a society that has failed? The University of California, Berkeley, Labor Center reports that half of all fast-food workers live on public assistance.[10] This same employment model is followed by nearly all the top-ten burger chains in the United States. See Table 5.1.

However, there are several emerging hamburger restaurants that are breaking out of the mold. See Table 5.2.

One such high-road restaurant is Moo Cluck Moo in Michigan, which owner Brian Parker opened with his business partner in April 2013. Parker's approach represents a wholly different business model than the low-road approach that is pervasive in the United States today.

Moo Cluck Moo's approach is centered on ensuring the highest quality of their primary output: hamburgers. To do so, the company sources all its beef from a farm in Ft. Wayne, Indiana, that utilizes authentic Japanese Kobe beef practices—methods of treating cows that ensure better, healthier, and more marbled beef. "[The farm] had a Kobe cattle farming master who sold them the [cattle] DNA, [who] was the architect of the grasses, forages, nutrients in the soil that they grow on their 200 acres." Cattle on the farm live at least three years in an open-range, antibiotic-free environment that takes every measure to ensure the animals live relatively stress-free. "I've walked the fields with these people," Parker says. "Their animals are happy, their tails are flipping, their coats are shiny; they're

Table 5.1 LOW-ROAD RESTAURANTS

	$10+ Wage for Non-tipped Workers	Hourly Wage for Tipped Workers Exceeds Minimum	Paid Sick Days	Promotion Practices	Stars
Burger King		n/a*		←	
Carl's Jr.		n/a*			
Five Guys Burgers and Fries		n/a*		←	
Jack in the Box		n/a*			
McDonald's		n/a*			
Red Robin		☺+			
Sonic Drive in		n/a*	—		
Wendy's		n/a*			
Whataburger		n/a*			
White Castle		n/a*			

*No tipped employees.

Table 5.2 HIGH-ROAD RESTAURANTS

	$10+ Wage for Non-tipped Workers	Hourly Wage for Tipped Workers Exceeds Minimum	Paid Sick Days	Promotion Practices	Stars
Black Star Co-op Austin, TX	💵	n/a*	🌡	←	★★
Fergie's Pub Philadelphia, PA	💵				
Grace Tavern Philadelphia, PA			🌡		
In-N-Out Burger National	💵	n/a*	🌡	←	★★
Monk's Café Philadelphia, PA			🌡		
Moo Cluck Moo Dearborn Heights, MI	💵	💲⁺	🌡	←	★★

(continued)

Table 5.2 CONTINUED

	$10+ Wage for Non-tipped Workers	Hourly Wage for Tipped Workers Exceeds Minimum	Paid Sick Days	Promotion Practices	Stars
Nodding Head Brewery *Philadelphia, PA*			🌡		
Rose Water *Brooklyn, NY*	💵		🌡		☆
Shake Shack *National*	💵	💲+		←	☆☆
The Belgian Café *Philadelphia, PA*			🌡		
The Local Table *Acton, MA*	💵	💲+		←	☆☆
Top Burger *Miami Beach, FL*		💲+	🌡	←	☆☆

*no tipped employees.

not listless, lifeless drugged animals. I think they're treated better than some humans."

Parker's experience being actively engaged with the sourcing of his restaurant's primary ingredient—a relatively uncommon experience among restaurant owners—has made the possibility of doing business any other way seem impossible. "These farmers are so into their product, its quality, the feeding process, the cattle life cycle," he says. "How could we not align with these people?"

Moo Cluck Moo's food sourcing practices dovetailed naturally into their employment practices. As Parker tells it, "We're not cutting bags open and just prepping everything; there's no processed food. We needed a higher caliber employee—not just to put the food together really well, but to do it consistently." To achieve excellence and continuity in his workforce, Parker has had to work upstream to create a work environment that was conducive to keeping people around. This entailed getting on board with the emerging national movement toward a universal $15 wage—only a slight increase over the $14 hourly rate that Moo Cluck Moo offered employees, but an important and symbolic one nonetheless.

For Parker and his partner, the benefits of their progressive approaches to business have been exponential. Their $15 wage announcement came in the midst of hundreds of fast-food-worker protests in the United States and around the world, and coincided with President Obama's visit to Michigan to campaign for increases in the minimum wage. Accordingly, Moo Cluck Moo's announcement that it would pay burger-making employees $15 an hour ended up providing the restaurant with a "year's amount of press, both local and national," according to Crain's Detroit.[11]

Parker recalls one bit of press with particular satisfaction. "I heard a staff member saying to a reporter, 'This isn't a job. A job is a means to an end. This is a career for me.'" Parker adds, "I want people to have a sense of place. They're putting their personal flag on our space, and it has to do with all the kinds of things I've been talking about. If you're sick, you're not going to get fired because you have the flu for two days. We want to be as humane as possible, because we don't have robots working in our facility. We want them to be stewards of the restaurant. They're killing it for us; we want to reward them."

THE LOW ROAD: MCDONALD'S

Brothers Richard and Maurice McDonald, known to their friends as Mac and Dick, opened their first drive-in restaurant, McDonald's Bar-B-Q, in 1940 with a $5,000 loan. McDonald's was their third business attempt; the brothers had previously attempted, unsuccessfully, to open a hot dog stand and a small movie theater. First-day sales at McDonald's were $366.12, with hamburgers selling at 15 cents each.[12] The restaurant did not become a success until eight years later, when the brothers overhauled their approach: they replaced a cast-iron grill with two six-foot grills, traded plates and silverware for paper goods, and reduced a large menu to a mere nine items–mostly burgers, fries, and shakes.[13]

The McDonalds' new approach caught the attention of a traveling salesman named Ray Kroc. Kroc's sales experience started in paper cups, then later expanded to a piece of kitchen equipment called the Multimixer, a milk-shake machine.[14] The device was popularized in part by a burger restaurant in San Bernadino, CA, which was booming with its "speedy service, low prices, and big volume" business model and its Multimixer-made milkshakes.[15] McDonald's, Kroc learned, used a fleet of eight Multimixers (at $150 a piece) to create up to 40 shakes at a time. Intrigued, Kroc flew to Los Angeles to find parking lots full of people ready to eat burgers, fries, and milkshakes. One customer explained to Kroc why he frequented the restaurant: "You'll get the best hamburger you ever ate for fifteen cents. And you don't have to wait and mess around tipping the waitress."[16] Kroc observed that customers varied from middle-aged men to younger women; the restaurant was kept immaculately clean; the menu was simple and to the point. He was sold; Kroc signed as McDonald's exclusive franchising agent and used his traveling salesman skills to open franchises across the United States.[17]

By 1956, there were fourteen McDonald's restaurants with sales totaling $1.2 million. By 1960, there were 228 restaurants with sales approximating $37.6 million. Five years later, 1965, saw 738 restaurants. Kroc eventually bought out the McDonald's brothers for $2.7 million.[18] As McDonald's began popping up all over the nation, the appeal was widespread; customers could purchase 15-cent hamburgers—a price at least 50 cents lower than most other competitors—and 12-cent French-fries.[19]

During the 1970s, McDonald's established itself and fast food as mainstays of American food consumption. As reported by *Corporate Rapsheet,* throughout this period, McDonald's continued to grow, "helped by demographic changes such as the migration of women into the waged labor market and by economic changes such as the sharp rise in the cost of food used to prepare meals at home. By spending large sums on marketing and advertising, the chains were able to turn fast-food "dining" into a socially acceptable way for a family to feed itself. Employing devices such as the Ronald McDonald character, McDonald's gained the loyalty of children, who became increasingly influential in determining where a family was going to eat out. In 1972, McDonald's reached $1 billion in total store sales and surpassed the U.S. Army as the nation's biggest dispenser of meals."[20]

McDonald's has grown into one of the most recognized global enterprises. The company has long prided itself on its size, and the scale of its operation has become part of its marketing lore: McDonald's feeds 23 million people daily in the United States; the company has over 31,000 stores in 118 countries.[21] They produce nine million pounds of french fries per day.[22] More Americans visit McDonald's than any other chain including Walmart; one in eight Americans have worked at McDonald's.[23]

Recent market changes may foretell trouble for McDonald's. In 2015 the company is expected to report its "first decline in domestic system-wide sales in at least thirty years, following a year of historically poor performance."[24] On the whole, customers seem to be visiting fast-food hamburger chains less. In January 2014, Don Thompson, then-McDonald's CEO admitted: "we've lost some of our customer relevance."[25] In particular, McDonald's sees itself losing customers to "healthier" fast-food options like Subway and Chipotle.

Working at McDonald's

McDonald's low wages and poor working conditions are beyond well known; they are a social touchstone for the understanding of poor working conditions. Less widely known is the lengths to which the company goes to lobby for lower wages and working conditions standards at the federal and state levels and squash any kind of dissent from its workforce or consumer base. A 1976 book on the company, *Big Mac: The Unauthorized Story of McDonald's*, reported that Ray Kroc was involved in numerous controversies regarding worker exploitation, including forcing employees to take lie detector tests and misappropriating their tips.[26] As early as 1972, Kroc was revealed for having donated $250,000 to Richard Nixon's 1972 re-election campaign, allegedly to push the Nixon Administration to get the "McDonald's bill" passed, which would have exempted students from the minimum wage.[27] In the 1970s and again in the 1990s, labor groups protested at McDonald's in San Francisco, Detroit, and Philadelphia, all over the company's low wages and lack of benefits.[28-29] Most recently, the national union Service Employees International Union (SEIU) has organized McDonald's and other fast-food workers as part of their campaign, Fast Food Forward, organizing one-day strikes and rallies in which they demand $15 an hour and a union.[30,31]

In a response to questions from press about whether he agreed that the minimum wage is difficult if not impossible to live on, former McDonald's CEO Don Thompson said that legislators would decide what to do about the minimum wage, and that the company would simply abide by any new legislation.[32] However, McDonald's has been engaged in lobbying against minimum wage increases for the last several decades.[33] As one of the top-four brands leading the NRA, McDonald's benefits from the NRA's active lobbying to prevent minimum wage, earned sick leave, and workers' rights legislation from passing, without having to sully the company brand by engaging in that lobbying directly.[34]

As a result of their poverty-level wages, most McDonald's employees receive their health coverage from Medicaid and other taxpayer-funded programs.[35] An October 2013 report by the National Employment Law Project (NELP) estimates that the public assistance provided to McDonald's workers in the United States costs $1.2 billion a year.[36] NELP reports that "McDonald's costs taxpayers nearly twice as much as its next-largest competitor, Yum! Brands."[37] Meanwhile, as McDonald's CEO, Donald Thompson was compensated nearly 13.7 million dollars before his retirement in 2015.[38]

The SEIU's Fast Food Forward campaign has raised and won several issues related to workers' rights at McDonalds's. In 2014, McDonald's workers in California, Michigan, and New York filed suit against the company and several franchise owners, charging them with forcing their employees to work off the clock and other overtime violations.[39]

The "workers claimed that their restaurants told them to show up to work, but then ordered them to wait an hour or two without pay until enough customers arrived." As a result of this lawsuit, several McDonald's franchisees and managers admitted to violations of the wages and hours laws. Kathryn Slater-Carter, franchisee owner of a McDonald's in Daly City, CA, admitted "she was encouraged by the company to cut employees' pay as a means of increasing her profits."[40] The problem, Slater-Carter claims, is that McDonald's tries to bring in customers through very low prices like the dollar hamburger and franchisees cannot keep up with such low values. So when Slater-Carter escalated her complaints to the corporate office, she claims the company representative said, "You guys can make more money if you pay your employees less."[41] Two former McDonald's store managers admitted to making their staff work without pay. Lakia Williams, a former assistant manager at a McDonald's in Charleston, SC, said she made adjustments to time sheets to avoid exceeding the company's strict limitations for labor costs.[42]

Finally, as part of the campaign, SEIU was able to get the U.S. National Labor Relations Board's (NLRB) Office of the General Counsel to issue complaints against McDonald's Corporation and some of its franchisees, claiming that they are responsible for seventy-eight cases of workers across the United States being "fired or intimidated for participating in union organizing and in a national protest movement calling for higher wages."[43]In a historic move impacting the future of franchising in America, the NLRB held that McDonald's could be held jointly liable for labor violations committed by its franchise operators.[44] In the past, McDonald's was shielded from the labor and employment law violations of its franchisees. In 2104, the NLRB ruled that McDonald's is a joint-employer because "McDonald's exercises so much influence over the restaurants telling them, with all sorts of requirements over how to cook, how to keep things clean, ways to handle" their employees. This means that McDonald's Corp. will be held jointly responsible for the actions of their franchisees.[45]

Throughout the last two years of SEIU-led strikes at McDonald's and other fast-food chains, McDonald's has been repeatedly questioned about how workers can survive on the wages the company pays. In response, McDonald's publicly issued an online budgeting tool for its workers, ostensibly to teach employees how to live on McDonald's wages. The tool was widely ridiculed as the 'McBudget'; commentators said that the tool "proved the fast-food giant pays its entry-level workers too little. The budget assumed that employees would need to get a second job just to earn a little more than $24,500 per year. The tool also left out essential expenses like food, water and clothing."[46] When asked if McDonald's is out of touch with what it's like to live on the minimum wage, former CEO Thompson responded that the website was intended to help those "entering the workforce for the first time or someone who really hasn't had financial planning or management practices or training, to be able to help manage finances."[47]

McDonald's has been the subject of numerous sexual harassment charges, and some of the most high-profile have involved teenage workers. The United States Equal Employment Opportunity Commisison (EEOC) asserts that teenage workers often experience violations of company antiharassment policies, procedures, and training programs because "in workplaces that commonly employ teens—fast-food restaurants, movie theaters, and retail stores—managers also often are teenagers."[48] In 2007, of 127 EEOC complaints involving teens dating back to 1999, seventy-two were against restaurant companies, and sixty-one of these complaints (85 percent) were based on sexual-harassment charges.[49]

The EEOC has filed a number of youth sexual-harassment cases against McDonald's and its largest franchisees owners. "In 2008

[McDonald's] franchisee JOBEC Inc. in Colorado paid $505,000 to settle such charges. In 2009 [McDonald's franchisee] LPG Enterprises in New Mexico paid $115,000. In 2012 [McDonald's franchisee] Missoula Mac Inc. in Wisconsin paid $1 million. In 2010 McDonald's itself had to pay $50,000 to settle similar harassment charges at one of its company-owned outlets in New Jersey."[50] In Colorado, a class of young female employees, age 15 to 17, filed suit against McDonald's franchises for being "subjected to egregious sexual harassment in the workplace by their male supervisor. The harassment allegedly included the supervisor biting the breasts and grabbing the buttocks of the class members, making numerous sexual comments, as well as offers of favors in exchange for sex."[51] In New Mexico, two young female employees filed suit for having been subjected to "egregious physical and verbal sexual harassment, including severe physical abuse."[52]In Wisconsin, a suit was filed against the owner and franchisee of twenty-five McDonald's restaurants for allowing male employees to engage in sexual harassment against young female workers, "including sexual comments, kissing, touching of their private areas, and forcing their hands onto the men's private parts."[53]

The Healthiness and Quality of the Big Mac

Few people think of McDonald's meals as healthy, high-quality meals. But the extent of healthy and safety problems with McDonald's food has been a source of controversy, especially when revelations emerge the company has misled consumers on these issues.

McDonald's faced litigation and ended up paying $10 million to settle after it came to light that French fries, which McDonald's claimed it was preparing with vegetable oil, were secretly prepared with beef flavoring.[54]After *Super Size Me*, in which filmmaker

Morgan Spurlock took the McDonald's challenge to eat nothing but McDonald's for a month, and suffered significant health consequences as a result, McDonald's introduced a new line of salads, announced plans to print nutrition data, and agreed to pay $8.5 million to settle a lawsuit alleging failure to inform the public about the presence of dangerous trans fats used.

The national consumers' organization Corporate Accountability International has been engaged in a multiyear campaign to stop McDonald's from marketing its unhealthy food—particularly through happy meals—to children. After pressure, McDonald's reduced portion size of of happy meals and added fruit.[55] During the 2013 shareholder meeting, 9-year-old Hannah Robertson confronted the former CEO Thompson about McDonald's marketing policies and asked why he was trying to "trick kids into eating food that isn't good for them by using toys and cartoon characters." His response was polite, thanking her for her question but said: "First off, we don't sell junk food, Hannah." Thompson then "went on to argue that his kids eat McDonald's and are healthy, adding that the chain has a plethora of healthy food options available on its menu."[56]

Even though McDonald's has aimed to change their image by marketing healthier food items, they recently (January 2015) re-introduced the triple cheeseburger to certain regions in the United States in the hopes of boosting sales, at least regionally.[57] In January 2015, it was reported that McDonald's Japan recalled one million McNuggets after at least two customers said they found plastic or vinyl fragments in their McNuggets.[58]

Case Study: Guadalupe's Story

Guadalupe is 38 years old and is a native of Orange County, California. She has worked at McDonald's since her separation two years ago, when the departure of her husband left her in care of the couple's daughter, who was seven at the time.

Guadalupe works more than forty hours per week to make ends meet, but says she hasn't always seen that money. "I used to work more than forty hours. I'm not sure if I got paid for all my hours." Guadalupe says she filed an administrative claim against the company for discrimination and retaliation after her manager mistreated her.

In her two years of working at McDonald's, Guadalupe has had to endure personal hardship and emotional pain, including moving her daughter to live with Guadalupe's ex-husband due to Guadalupe's insufficient income. "It's been so bad, so little money. With my schedule—I work 4 or 5 A.M. to 12 or 1 in afternoon, it's tough to find a babysitter, someone who I can trust to leave my daughter with. Has to be someone I trust. I try to see her often. [Her father] brings her to me. I drive to where they are, and we play, or go to park, or go to movies, but not very often."

Guadalupe has frequently worked while sick at McDonald's. "All of us have. People are sick with flu in the kitchen, working like that. I work the drive-through window, and I take orders in the rain."

Guadalupe recently became involved with the Fight for 15—a collective movement of fast-food workers across the United States fighting for a livable wage for all workers. She spoke with a recruiter, and her experience since then has changed her goals from personal to something more collective. "I fell in love with this organization, this fight; all that matters is to join this fight to help my other co-workers. I've been working for two-and-a-half years, but others have been working for ten, twelve, fifteen years."

Guadalupe has encountered a lot of fear among other McDonald's workers who share their challenges in the company with her but are unwilling—as of yet—to join the fight out of fear of retaliation. Employees will share specific grievances, but will stop short of escalating. "There's a woman in her fifties who's been at McDonald's for twelve years. She burned herself cleaning the oil fryers, from her elbow to the tip of her fingers, really badly. I felt pain when I saw her arm. I told her I want to try to help her, to engage her with the union, so she can fight. She didn't even go to the doctor for the burn. She just put ointment on and she continued working that day." Without the right to earned sick leave, Guadalupe reports that McDonald's workers like this woman regularly keep working when injured. "She's not doing anything to change it. It's a lot of thinking she might get fired. Retaliation is against the law, but [she wouldn't pursue it]."

Guadalupe looks forward to winning the campaign. "Once I get $15 and a union, I want to get myself in college, build a career. I'll be an organizer, start fighting for people to get a union."

THE HIGH ROAD: IN-N-OUT BURGER

In-N-Out Burger was founded in 1948 by Esther and Harry Snyder in Baldwin Park, California. Esther Snyder (nee Johnson) was born in 1920 to a family of coalminers. Even though her parents knew that their opportunities were limited due to their modest circumstances, they emphasized the importance of school, and Esther excelled academically, eventually going to college to study elementary school education. After graduation, she became a schoolteacher; then, during World War II, she went on to enlist in the navy's newly created (and somewhat controversial) Women Accepted for Voluntary Emergency Service (WAVES) program. Through this program she contributed to the war effort by serving as a surgical nurse and pharmacist's mate over a span of three years.[59]

Harry Snyder, the son of Dutch immigrants, was born on September 9, 1913 in Canada. At 2 years old, his family emigrated

135

from Canada to Seattle. His father Hendrick Snyder worked as a painter, and his mother Mary worked as a housecleaner. Harry describes his father as a "die-hard socialist" who strongly believed in entrepreneurialism and redistribution of wealth."[60] In the 1920s when Seattle's economy was facing a downturn, Hendrick moved to Los Angeles, CA and eventually brought over the rest of the family. Hendrick continued to work as a painter and Mary continued working as a housekeeper. Eventually Hendrick lost his job and his family relied solely on Mary's income until Harry, at approximately 15 years of age, began taking odd jobs as a paperboy, grocery store worker, selling sandwiches, and delivering food. [61] Harry describes himself during high school as a communist who thought "we needed a whole new system" where everyone would work together ands share everything "instead of some getting it all." [62] Harry was shaped by "watching his parents labor to provide for his family, chasing one opportunity after another." [63] Biographer Stacy Perman explains that "perhaps as a result of Harry's brief flirtation with communism and his disgust for economic inequity, he always exhibited a soft spot for those in need."[64]

Going Their Own Way

By 1947, at age 34, Harry had met Esther, who was a restaurant manager at the time.

Despite a few failed attempts to open other small businesses, Harry was motivated to start a hamburger stand that would cater to an increasingly mobile population. Short on cash, he partnered with Charles Noddin who would help finance the venture with $5,000.[65] Harry also sought business advice from Carl N. Karcher, who, at the time, was the founder of a small, but growing chain called Carl's Jr.[66] Karcher describes the Snyders as being "very particular about their people smiling . . . they wanted their employees to feel like they were part of the company, like they were owners themselves."[67]

In-N-Out has remained a family-owned restaurant since it started.[68] The Snyder's basic philosophy and approach to their restaurant was "healthy food, hard work, accessibility to travelers, low prices, consistent ethics and values, and organic growth that preserves company culture."[69]

By the time Harry died from cancer in 1976, In-N-Out had grown to eighteen drive-throughs in Los Angeles County.[70] At this point ownership passed to his son Rich Snyder, 24 years old at the time. Their other son, Guy Snyder was 25 and became the executive vice-president. It was Rich who, with his mother, became a passionate Christian at Calvary Chapel, and began putting the Bible references on the bottom inside lip of the restaurant's beverage cups.[71] Rich was president until his death in a 1993 plane crash. His brother Guy inherited the business. Unfortunately, according to Stacy Perman's book on the company, Guy's lifestyle revolved around car racing and substance use, and he was not able to contribute to the company's functioning or success.[72] As a result, Esther returned to take control until her death in 2006, after which her granddaughter Lynsi Torres, daughter of Guy Snyder, then took over the company as the sole remaining heir.[73] Lynsi is currently the president and half-owner and will become the full owner when she is 35.[74]

In-N-Out currently employs four thousand workers and enjoys approximately $625 million in sales annually, according to *Bloomberg*.[75] Serving hamburgers, cheeseburgers, the Double-Double (two patties and two slices of cheese), and French fries, In-N-Out does not franchise restaurants. It follows a slow growth model, opening approximately ten new locations each year. The company has restaurants in five states: California, Arizona, Nevada, Texas, and Utah, with plans to expand to Florida. The company does not venture out too far away from its headquarters in

California to maintain strict control over food and service quality throughout its chain.[76]

The company is known for its secrecy—as a private family company, there is not much information made publicly available, and its leadership rarely grants interviews.[77] Stacy Perman was the only person ever granted such interviews, and wrote a book on the company on that basis in 2009. Even within the restaurant industry, few have met or know much about Lynsi Torres, the sole In-N-Out heir.[78] Currently in her early 30s, she is one of the youngest female billionaires in the world.[79]

Working at In-N-Out

In-N-Out is distinguished by its higher-than-average worker pay.[80] When Glassdoor ranked In-N-Out number eight in its list of top-ten places to work based on employee feedback, the *Huffington Post* reported, "In an industry known for low salaries and poor treatment of workers In-N-Out is often recognized for playing against type . . . the starting wage at the company is $10.50 an hour. That's a lot higher than the median hourly pay for fast-food workers nationwide, which is $8.94 an hour."[81]

In addition to its higher starting wage, In-N-Out offers part-time and full-time employees benefits that include flexible schedules to accommodate school and other activities, paid vacations, free meals, comprehensive training, and a 401k plan.[82] Full-time associates and their dependents are offered medical insurance, dental insurance, vision care, life insurance, business and travel insurance, 401k, holiday pay, free meals on workdays, 15 percent discounts at the store, vacation days, and six sick days per year. Part-time associates are offered all of the above except medical care, with vacation and sick pay being pro-rated based on hours. Assistant store managers earn between

$40,000 and $70,000 annually, and store managers can make over $100,000.[83]

Biographer Stacy Perman writes that these conditions are not new. "From the very beginning, Harry offered his workers the opportunity to build a career . . . While everyone had to start at the bottom . . . everyone was also given the opportunity to advance."[84] Years ahead of the curve, Harry "gave his associates a measure of ownership in the enterprise and he remunerated them handsomely for their ability to meet their targets and surpass them."[85] In 1989 part-time associates earned $6 per hour, well above the minimum wage of $4.25. Managers made an average of $63,000 annually.[86] In 2006, In-N-Out paid workers $9.50, whereas the California minimum wage was $6.50.[87] Perman writes that "The Snyders displayed an uncommon respect for their workers . . . they never looked at their workers as just employees but saw them as part of their growing, extended family the Snyders made sure to know each individual by name . . . they banished the words 'employees' and 'workers' altogether and instead referred to them strictly as 'associates.' The result was that from the outset, In-N-Out had the feel not of a workplace but of a joint enterprise in which everyone shared."[88] In 1988, when California raised its minimum wage, the *Orange County Register* "called Rich Snyder perhaps the only restaurant executive in the state to favor a widespread pay hike."[89]

In an interview, company Vice President Carl Van Fleet explained that, as a result of higher wages and better benefits, "we do enjoy relatively low turnover and that, of course, leads to a more experienced team working in our restaurants. The raises that our associates earn for mastering different positions makes it possible for them to earn more as they gain that experience."[90] "We strive to create a working environment that is upbeat, enthusiastic and customer-focused," Van Fleet wrote in an email to The Huffington Post. "A higher pay structure is helpful in making that happen, but it is only part of our approach. It is equally important to treat our associates well and maintain that positive working environment in all of our restaurants."[91]

Food Quality

In his book *Fast Food Nation*, Eric Schlosser offered approval and praise to only one fast-food company: In-N-Out Burger.[92] "The chain famously does not use microwaves, heat lamps, or freezers, and it has no franchise operators."[93]High-quality food has been key to In-N-Out's model from the beginning. Harry Snyder was known as being "fanatical about quality," inspecting everything that was used in his restaurant, and frequently visited his meat suppliers.[94] While other fast food joints were adding chemicals, additives, and coloring agents to the food they were serving, in "Harry's mind, there was just no substitute for the real thing. All hamburgers were made from fresh, 100 percent additive-, filler-, and preservative-free beef ...[and fries were] cooked in cholesterol-free, 100 percent vegetable oil .... In-N-Out refused to use anything but 100 percent ice cream in their milkshakes."[95]

Hamburger buns at In-N-Out are made from sponge dough, a type of bread that takes longer and uses relatively few ingredients.[96] Burgers are made from 100 percent beef; they are never frozen.[97] Stores receive deliveries every other day to make sure there is always fresh produce. The company chooses to spend more than other fast-food restaurant companies to ensure freshness.[98]

The Orange County Register attributes the company's slow, measured growth to these imperatives of quality and practice:

"Slow growth, a hallmark of the company's operations since the beginning, is a side-effect of its commitment to serve only high-quality, fresh food."[99]

NOTES

1. Micaela Pantke, "Antique Roman Dishes – Collection," Carnegie Mellon School of Computer Science Recipe Archive, Carnegie Mellon University, (accessed September 26, 2014).
2. Alan Beardsworth, Teresa Keil, *Sociology on the Menu: An Invitation to the Study of Food and Society*, (New York: Routledge, 1997)..
3. Leslie Page Moch, *Moving Europeans: Migration in Western Europe Since 1650* (2nd ed.). (Bloomington: Indiana University Press, 2003).
4. Josh Ozersky, *The Hamburger: A History (Icons of America)* (London: Yale University Press, 2008).
5. N. A. M. Rodger, *The Insatiable Earl: A Life of John Montagu, Fourth Earl of Sandwich 1718–1792* (W W Norton & Co Inc., 1994), 480.
6. Andrew F. Smith, *Hamburger: A Global History* (London: Reaktion Books, 2008.)
7. Myron Heuer, "The Real Home of the Hamburger." *Herald & Journal*, October 12, 1999. <http://www.herald-journal.com/archives/1998/columns/mh101298.html>
8. Liz Alderman and Steven Greenhouse, "Living Wages, Rarity for U.S. Fast-Food Workers, Served Up in Denmark," *The New York Times*, October 27, 2014, http://www.nytimes.com/2014/10/28/business/international/living-wages-served-in-denmark-fast-food-restaurants.html.
9. Ibid.
10. S. A. Allegretto, M. Doussard, D. Graham-Squire, K. Jacobs, D. Thompson, and J. Thompson. *Fast Food, Poverty Wages: The Public Cost of Low-Wage Jobs in the Fast-Food Industry.* (Berkeley: UC Berkeley Center for Labor Research and Education, 2013).
11. http://www.crainsdetroit.com/article/20130911/blog006/130919957/moo-cluck-moos-15-an-hour-story-starts-with-a-lesson-in-minimum-wage
12. "Beyond the Golden Arches: Inside McDonald's." *Bloomberg.com*. <http://www.bloomberg.com/video/beyond-the-golden-arches-inside-mcdonald-s-08-01-Mlmx~rYMTdGO_UwpzkT8ng.html>.
13. Stacy Perman,. *In-N-Out Burger: A Behind-the-counter Look at the Fast-food Chain That Breaks All the Rules.* (New York: Collins Business, 2009). 46–47.
14. Kroc, Ray. *Grinding It Out: The Making of McDonald's.* New York, NY: St. Martin's Press, 1987, p.6.
15. Patricia Sowell Harris,. *None of Us Is as Good as All of Us: How McDonald's Prospers by Embracing Inclusion and Diversity.* (Hoboken, NJ: John Wiley & Sons, 2009). 15.
16. Kroc, 7.
17. Ibid.; Harris, 16–17.
18. Harris, 19.

19. Joe L. Kincheloe, *The Sign of the Burger: McDonald's and the Culture of Power.* (Philadelphia: Temple University Press, 2002) 54.

20. Corporate Research Rap Sheet: McDonald's, http://www.corp-research. org/corporaterapsheets, October 13, 2014.

21. Karen Feridun, "Origins: McDonald's Hamburger," Side Dish, GoIndie. com, August 20, 2010, http://www.goindie.com/dish/index.cfm/origins/ article/id/19582A04-7B59-4464-9073B7CB1AD90478.

22. William Harris, "10 Most Popular McDonald's Menu Items of All Time" HowStuffWorks.com, April 7, 2009, http://money.howstuffworks.com/ 10-popular-mcdonalds-menu-items.htm.

23. Gus Lubin, "13 Disturbing Facts About McDonald's," *The Fiscal Times*, April 30, 2012, http://www.thefiscaltimes.com/Articles/2012/04/30/ 13-Disturbing-Facts-About-McDonalds.

24. Jonathan Maze,. "McDonald's 2014 Performance May be Worst in Decades." *Nation's Restaurant News*, January 15, 2015. <http://nrn.com/corporate-news/mcdonald-s-2014-performance-may-be-worst-decades?page=1>.

25. Jillian Berman, "Can This Guy Save McDonald's" *Huffington Post*, August 22, 2014. <http://www.huffingtonpost.com/2014/08/22/mcdonalds-us-president_n_5699256.html>.

26. Eric Pace,. "Ray A. Kroc Dies at 81-- Built McDonald's Chain." *The New York Times*, Jan. 15, 1984.

27. John F. Love, *McDonald's: Behind the Arches.* (New York: Bantam, 1986),. 357.

28. Philip.Mattera, "McDonald's: Corporate Rap Sheet." *Corporate Research*, October 13, 2014. <http://www.corp-research.org/mcdonalds>.

29. Ibid.

30. Ibid.

31. Ibid.

32. Phil Rosenthal, "CEO: McDonald's would 'manage' minimum wage hike," *Chicago Tribune*, May 25, 2014, http://articles.chicagotribune.com/2014-05-25/business/ct-rosenthal-mcdonalds-wage-0525-biz-20140525_1_minimum-wage-chief-executive-don-thompson-mcdonald.

33. Eric Schlosser, *Fast Food Nation: The Dark Side of the All-American Meal* (New York: Houghton Mifflin Company, 2001), 37.

34. Steven Rosenthal, "The Other NRA: How the Insidiously Powerful Restaurant Lobby Makes Sure Fast-Food Workers Get Poverty Wages and Have to Work While Sick," Alternet, August 27, 2013, http://www.alternet. org/labor/other-nra-how-insidiously-powerful-restaurant-lobby-makes-sure-fast-food-workers-get-poverty.

35. "Hidden Tax Payer Costs: Disclosures of Employers Whose Workers and Their Dependents are Using State Health Insurance Programs." *Good Jobs First.*

http://www.goodjobsfirst.org/corporate-subsidy-watch/hidden-taxpayer-costs (accessed July 24, 2013); Mattera,. "McDonald's: Corporate Rap Sheet."

36. Data Brief. "Super-sizing Public Costs: How Low Wages at Top Fast-Food Chains Leave Taxpayers Footing the Bill." National Employment Law Project (NELP). October 2013.

37. Ibid.

38. Ibid.

39. Steven Greenhouse,. "McDonald's Workers File Wage Suits in 3 States." *The New York Times.* March 13, 2014.

40. Hayley Peterson, "McDonald's Franchisee Claims Company Encouraged Her to Cut Employee Pay." *Business Insider,* August 4, 2014. <http://www.businessinsider.com/mcdonalds-franchisee-complaint-2014-8>.

41. Ibid.

42. Hayley Peterson,. "McDonald's Managers Admit to Making Staff Work Without Pay." *Business Insider,* April 2, 2014. <http://www.businessinsider.com/mcdonalds-managers-withheld-pay-2014-4>.

43. Daniel Wiessner, "U.S. Labor Agency Files Complaints Against McDonald's." *Reuters,* December 19, 2014.

44. Steven Greenhouse, "McDonald's Ruling Could Open Door for Unions." *The New York Times.* July 29, 2014.

45. Hari Sreenivasan, & Steven Greenhouse. "McDonald's Charged With Abusing Workers Over Wage Protests." *PBS,* December 21, 2014.

46. Caroline.Fairchild, "McDonalds' CEO: We've 'Always Been An Above-Minimum Wage Employer.'" *Huffington Post,* July 24, 2013. <http://www.huffingtonpost.com/2013/07/24/mcdonalds-minimum-wage_n_3644081.html>.

47. "Beyond the Golden Arches: Inside McDonald's." *Bloomberg.com.* Bloomberg. <http://www.bloomberg.com/video/beyond-the-golden-arches-inside-mcdonald-s-08-01-Mlmx~rYMTdGO_UwpzkT8ng.html>.

48. Jill Schachner Chanen, "New Troubles for Teens at Work." *ABA Journal* 22 (2008). <http://www.abajournal.com/magazine/article/new_troubles_for_teens_at_work>

49. Ibid.

50. Mattera,. "McDonald's: Corporate Rap Sheet."

51. "McDonald's Franchise to Pay $505,000 for Sexual Harassment of Young Women, Including Teens." The U.S. Equal Employment Opportunity Commission. April 7, 2008. <http://www.eeoc.gov/eeoc/newsroom/release/archive/4-7-08.html>.

52. "McDonald's Franchise to Pay $115,000 for Sexual Harassment of Two Young Women." The U.S. Equal Employment Opportunity Commission. March 24, 2009. <http://www.eeoc.gov/eeoc/newsroom/release/archive/3-24-09c.html>.

53. "Owner of 25 McDonald's Restaurants to Pay $1 Million in EEOC Sexual Harassment Suit." The U.S. Equal Employment Opportunity Commission. July 18, 2012. <http://www.eeoc.gov/eeoc/newsroom/release/7-18-12a.cfm>.

54. Laurie Goodstein, "For Hindus and Vegetarians, Surprise in McDonald's Fries." *The New York Times,* May 20, 2001.

55. Stephanie Strom,. "McDonald's Trims Its Happy Meal." *The New York Times,* July 26, 2011.

56. Meredith Bennett-Smith, "'We Don't Sell Junk Food:' McDonald's CEO Responds to 9-Year-Old Critic Hannah Robertson. *Huffington Post,* May 30, 2013. <http://www.huffingtonpost.com/2013/05/30/we-dont-sell-junk-food-mcdonalds-ceo-hannah-robertson_n_3360668.html>.

57. Bruce Horovitz,. "McDonald's Triple Cheeseburger Returns." *USA Today,* January 15, 2015. <http://www.usatoday.com/story/money/2015/01/15/mcdonalds-triple-cheeseburger-fast-food-restaurants-food/21803715/>.

58. Julia Lurie, "McDonald's Just Recalled 1 Million Chicken McNuggets for a Super-Gross Reason." *Mother Jones,* January 15, 2015. <http://www.motherjones.com/blue-marble/2015/01/mcdonalds-just-recalled-one-million-chicken-mcnuggets-super-gross-reason>.

59. Stacy Perman, *In-N-Out Burger: A Behind-the-Counter Look at the Fast-food Chain That Breaks All the Rules.* (New York: Collins Business, 2009). 24–26.

60. Ibid., 16–17.

61. Ibid., 19.

62. Ibid., 20.

63. Ibid., 19.

64. Ibid.. 81.

65. Ibid., 33.

66. Ibid., 35.

67. Ibid., 37.

68. David W. Gill, *Media Reviews: In-n-Out Burger: A Behind-the-Counter Look at the Fast-Food Chain That Breaks All the Rules by Stacy Perman,* EthixBiz, 2009. <http://ethixbiz.com/wp-content/uploads/2015/08/Perman-S.-In-n-Out-Burger.pdf>

69. Perman, Stacy. *In-N-Out Burger: A Behind-the-counter Look at the Fast-food Chain That Breaks All the Rules.* New York: Collins Business, 2009. Print, p. 12

70. Rick Paulas, "Lynsi Torres, the 30-Year-Old Owner of In-N-Out." *KCET,* Feb. 4, 2013. <http://www.kcet.org/living/food/food-rant/lynsi-torres-the-30-year-old-owner-of-in-n-out.html>; Richard Clough, "Drag-Racing Heiress Keeps In-N-Out on Course," *OC Register,* Feb. 22, 2013. <http://www.ocregister.

com/articles/torres-496945-company-snyder.html>; Company profile, http://www.fundinguniverse.com/company-histories/in-n-out-burger-history/.

71. Gill, *Media Reviews: In-n-Out Burger*

72. Ibid.

73. Paulas, Rick. "Lynsi Torres,; Richard Clough, "Drag-Racing Heiress; Company profile,.

74. Ibid.

75. Seth Lubove. "Youngest American Women Billionaire Found With In-N-Out." *Bloomberg*, Feb. 4, 2013.

76. In-N-Out Company Profile. Hoover's Company Records, In-depth Records, December 23, 2014. LexisNexis Academic. <http://www.lexisnexis.com/hottopics/lnacademic/>

77. Gill, Review, *In-n-Out Burger*

78. Lubove, "Youngest American Women Billionaire."

79. Paula Forbes, "Meet Lynsi Torres, In-N-Out's Billionaire Burger Heiress." *Eater*, Feb. 4, 2013. <http://www.eater.com/2013/2/4/6485413/meet-lynsi-torres- in-n-outs-billionaire-burger-heiress>

80. Gill, *Media Reviews: In-n-Out Burger*

81. Emily Cohn, "In-N-Out Ranks Higher Than Facebook and Apple on New List of Best Places to Work." *The Huffington Post*, December 10, 2014. <http://www.huffingtonpost.com/2014/12/10/in-n-out-best-jobs-glassdoor_n_6284568.html>.

82. In-N-Out Website: http://www.in-n-out.com/employment/restaurant.aspx

83. Ashley Lutz, "In-N-Out Employees Can Work Their Way Up To $120,000 A Year With No Degree or Previous Experience." *Business Insider*, Feb. 27, 2013. <http://www.businessinsider.com/in-and-out-employee-pay-2013-2>.

84. Perman, 54.

85. Perman, 54.

86. Company History: http://www.fundinguniverse.com/company-histories/in-n-out-burger-history/

87. Perman, 139.

88. Perman, 55.

89. Perman, 138.

90. Rick Paulas, "Why Does In-N-Out Pay So Well?" *KCET*, October 16, 2013. <http://www.kcet.org/living/food/food-rant/why-does-in-n-out-pay-so-well.html>.

91. Cohn, "In-N-Out Ranks Higher Than Facebook and Apple."

92. Gill, *Media Reviews: In-n-Out Burger*

93. In-N-Out Company Profile. Hoover's Company Records.

94. Perman, 44.
95. Perman, 90.
96. *California's Gold #146: In-N-Out Burger. California's Gold,* 2010. Huell Howser Productions, 2010. <http://vimeo.com/36550339>.
97. Ibid.
98. Ibid.
99. Gill, *Media Reviews: In-n-Out Burger*

[6]

A TALE OF TWO SANDWICHES

The American sandwich shop has become a dominating segment of the restaurant industry. Today, Subway has surpassed McDonald's in the number of stores they have worldwide,[1] and like other chain restaurants, sandwich shops have come to follow the "race to the bottom" standards of the National Restaurant Association. See Table 6.1.

This chapter is the tale of two sandwich shops. Both shops were started by two white males, both started small in smalltown America. But the similarities end there. This is the story of two very different patterns of growth—one a very careful, thoughtful, planned vision of growth and the other focused on rapid replication.

Of course, sandwich shops do not intrinsically have to provide low wages and poor benefits. Several of our high-road employer partners provide quality sandwiches and also fare quite well on raises, benefits, and promotions. See Table 6.2.

THE LOW ROAD: SUBWAY: THE FASTEST GROWING SANDWICH CHAIN IN THE WORLD

In 1965, Fred DeLuca was a 17-year-old college student in Bridgeport Connecticut looking for a way to pay for medical school.

Table 6.2 LOW-ROAD RESTAURANTS

	$10+ Wage for Non-Tipped Workers	Hourly Wage for Tipped Workers Exceeds Minimum	Paid Sick Days	Promotion Practices	Stars
Arby's		n/a*			
Firehouse Subs		n/a*			
Jason's Deli		n/a*		←	
Jersey Mike's Subs	💲				
Jimmy John's Gourmet Sandwiches		n/a*			
McAlister's Deli		n/a*		←	
Potbelly Sandwiches		n/a*			
Quiznos Subs		n/a*			
Schlotzksy's		n/a*			
Subway		n/a*			

*No tipped employees.

Table 6.1 HIGH-ROAD RESTAURANTS

	$10+ Wage for Non-Tipped Workers	Hourly Wage for Tipped Workers Exceeds Minimum	Paid Sick Days	Promotion Practices	Stars
Bob's Clam Hut *Kittery, ME*		💲+		←	★
Russell St. Deli *Detroit, MI*	💵			←	★★
The Sandwich Hut *Providence, RI*	💵		🌡	←	★★
West Avenue Café *Miami Beach, FL*	💵			←	★
Zingerman's Roadhouse *Ann Arbor, MI*	💵		🌡	←	★★

DeLuca had grown up in a public housing project in the Bronx, New York, and his family did not have enough money to further his education. A family friend, Dr. Peter Buck, suggested he open a sandwich shop to generate the cash, and gave him $1000 to start the company. They called it Pete's Super Submarines.[2,3]

Pete's would later become Subway, the fastest growing sandwich shop in the world. Fred was focused from the outset on growth. "We didn't have any big thought process except that, 'ok, franchising will help us get to our goal of 32 stores and help us run stores farther away from home.'" But when they reached that goal, 32 stores seemed small. "Could we open as many stores as McDonald's had everywhere? I thought, 'Yeah, why not? Anywhere they have a store, we can have a store.'"

DeLuca became a pioneer—or at least a titan—in restaurant franchising. "I tell everybody there are only three things that we do. We build sales at the store level, we build profits at the store level, and we build more stores."[4]

Fred did indeed meet and surpass his goal of being everywhere McDonald's is. Subway surpassed the McDonalds store count in the United States in 2002, then globally in 2010.[5] Subway is now the largest restaurant chain in the world, with 44,020 stores in 110 countries.[6]

It is notable that Fred's list of three things that Subway does did *not* include making a quality sandwich. The company's central marketing campaign focuses on "Eat Fresh," the idea that the restaurants provide fresh ingredients to form a healthy, low-calorie meal; the restaurants have baked their own bread in the store since 1983.[7,8] Many remember Jared "The Subway Guy" Fogle, who served as Subway's emblem of fresh and healthy eating because he reportedly lost 245 pounds in one year by replacing his meals with Subway Sandwiches.[9,10] Jared's rise to fame was inspired by Subway's "7 under 6," seven subs with 6 grams of fat or less.[11] Since

2011 Subway has worked to reduce sodium in their sandwiches due to their concern for hypertension and heart disease.[12] However, the rapid growth model has had mixed results with regard to providing fresh and healthy food.

On the one hand, Subway touts the awards it has received from animal rights and environmental groups. The animal welfare group Compassion Over Killing has conducted a campaign called "WeLoveSubway," advocating for more vegan options at Subway. As a result, Subway stores in Canada, Los Angeles, and the Washington DC metropolitan area now offer up to four vegan sandwiches.[13] Two large animal-welfare groups, People for the Ethical Treatment of Animals and The Humane Society, have praised Subway for their commitment to the humane treatment of animals. Subway in the United Kingdom does not use gestation crates for sows, and, as of 2013, in Europe, it uses only free range eggs for breakfast omelets.[14]

Subway has also demonstrated a commitment to environmental sustainability. The restaurant company opened its first Leadership in Energy and Environmental Design (LEED)-certified building in 2007. Subway has opened fourteen "Eco-Restaurants" since then, featuring low-flow faucets, energy-efficient lighting, recycled packing materials, and compost where possible.[15,16]

Eating Fresh?

On the other hand, Subway's central marketing campaign called "Eat Fresh," focused on eating fresh and healthy meals, has not always lived up to its name. A number of studies have compared the eating habits of customers at McDonalds and Subway and found that people consumed similar amounts of calories at both stores.[17] Despite Subway offering healthy sandwich options, often costumers purchased high calorie sodas, cookies, chips, and underestimated their calorie intake.[18] The UK Daily Mail reports that some Subway sandwiches have more calories and salt than a Big Mac.[19]

In August 2014, a dispute erupted between a former Australian Subway Franchisee owner, Arun Singhal, and Subway Corporation. Singhal claimed that he approached the corporation regarding the misleading "six grams of fat or less" advertising, and that the corporation retaliated against him in a way that eventually led to the closure of his Subway store.[20] Due to the dispute, Singhal threatened to leak a video with information about the misleading campaign. In response, Subway obtained a restraining order blocking the release of any information regarding Subway's business practices.[21] The video was finally released. It demonstrated how fine print under Subway's "six grams of fat or less" claim reads: "Energy values refer to Subs prepared on white bread according to standard recipes. Customer requests to modify standard recipe may increase energy values." The fine print includes an asterisked notation: "Regular Subway Six Inch sub with 6 grams of fat or less prepared to standard recipe on white bread without cheese or additional non-low-fat condiments such as mayonnaise."[22]

Many customers request sauce and cheese on their sandwiches, and also ask for different types of bread, increasing their calorie intake.[23] Thus, Singhal claimed that the "six grams of fat or less" misleads customers about how many calories and grams of fat they are actually consuming.

A high-profile scandal broke in February 2014 when food blogger and activist Vani Hari gathered more than 50,000 signatures on a petition demanding that Subway remove a chemical called azodicarbonamide from its breads.[24] Azodicarbonamide is most often used to 'increase elasticity in everything from yoga mats to shoe rubber to synthetic leather'.[25] Subway used the chemical to whiten its bread dough and allow sandwich bread to bake more quickly; in April 2014, they announced that they would remove the chemical, though Subway denied it was a result of the food blogger's efforts.[26] Azodicarbonamide is legal in the United States and has been approved by the U.S. Department of Agriculture and the U.S. Food and Drug Administration (FDA). However, the chemical has been banned in Europe and Australia, where experts at the World Health Organization published a report suggesting that azodicarbonamide can cause asthma when used in an industrial setting, and the United Kingom includes it in its "List of substances that can cause occupational asthma."[27,28] In addition, Subway's 9-grain wheat, white, and sourdough breads are still conditioned with chemicals like sodium stearoyl lactylate and ammonium sulfate.[29]

As alarming as the quality of Subway's ingredients are questions about its food safety. In 2014, a norovirus outbreak in a Subway Restaurant in Colorado left twenty people sick.[30] Between 2007 and 2012, fifty-five New York Subway stores were closed by the City Health Department for health code violations, including rodent infestations and poor refrigeration.[31] More Subway stores were closed in New York than any other franchise in that time frame.[32] In 2010, at least ninety-seven people were diagnosed with salmonella poisoning.[33] This was the second outbreak Subway restaurants in Illinois faced in 2010; several months earlier, seventy-eight people fell ill during a shigellosis outbreak.[34,35]

As discussed elsewhere in this book, food safety problems are exacerbated by sick workers. Of the more than 5,000 restaurant workers surveyed by ROC United, 90 percent reported not having paid sick days, and two-thirds reported cooking, preparing, and serving food while sick.[36] Subway does not provide earned sick leave to its workers. On the contrary, as a member of the National Restaurant Association, Subway has paid for lobbyists who have succeeded in passing legislation in twelve states to preemptively prohibit citizens from passing local earned sick leave ordinances, even if they democratically decide to do so.[37]

On July 11, 2014, in Freeport, Texas, Subway employee Elizabeth Taff says she was forced to continue to work while suffering from a stomach illness and, ultimately, was fired the same day. She vomited several times during her shift, but the manager refused to let her leave unless she could find someone to cover her shift. Taff went outside behind the restaurant and employees at a nearby business called an ambulance when they saw her reeling on the ground. Taff was officially fired for "poor performance and insubordination" but recalls her boss saying, "if you can't handle working while feeling ill you don't need to work here."[38] Another worker called the ambulance and posted photos on Facebook captioned: "If you planned on eating Freeport Subway today I advise not to, I witnessed an employee vomiting and her manager telling her to just switch shirts."[39] Fortunately, a growing movement has passed earned-sick-leave legislation in four states and in over nineteen cities nationwide,[40] and the Obama White House has indicated its support of earned-sick-leave legislation.[41]

What Rapid Growth Means for Workers and Franchisees

Subway's advertising describes Subway employees as sandwich artists. By paying them the minimum wage, they make a strong statement on the value of the "art" their employees create.[42] The results of these pay practices? Taxpayers pay $436 million annually in public assistance to Subway employees.[43] Furthermore, Subway franchisees have been found in violation of the law with regard to properly paying their employees even the meager minimum wage. From 2000 to 2013, Subway franchisees were found in violation of wage and hour rules in more than 1,100 investigations. The combined investigations total about "17,000 Fair Labor Standards Act violations and resulted in franchisees having to reimburse Subway workers more than $3.8 million over the years."[44] Subway is somewhat unique in wage and hour violations. The total number of violations at Subway "was far greater than the next highest fast food offenders: McDonald's and Dunkin' Donuts."[45]

The offenses have been significant. A Minnesota Subway franchisee that failed to pay minimum wages and shaved hours from employees' time records had to pay sixteen workers a total of $9,800 in back wages."[46] An Ohio Subway franchisee who owned five Subway restaurants, was sued for both overtime and child labor laws by the Department of Labor. Sixty-eight workers were asked to stay after the restaurants closed to finish nightly closing procedures, but were not paid for their time. The franchise company "also violated the FLSA's Hazardous Occupations Order No. 12, which prohibits workers under age 18 from loading, operating or unloading paper balers or trash compactors. Five minors employed by Hray Enterprises were required to load and operate two paper balers and one trash compactor on a regular basis."[47]

Subway's wage and hour violations were serious enough to motivate the U.S. Department of Labor to seek to partner with Subway headquarters to increase legal compliance.[48] To his credit, Subway's CEO Fred de Luca indicated willingness to work with the Department of Labor to make course correction, but blamed the scope of the company's illegal activity on the size of the company and the franchise model—which many claim he has promulgated more than any other corporate leader. "First of all, the fact that we have so many stores has an impact on how many violations there are. If we had 5,000 stores, there would be a smaller number than if we had 25,000 . . . The vast majority of our owners are doing the right thing but some are not. I would say this: We, as a company, realize that some of our owners have not done the right thing."[49]

Until recently, Subway was not liable for individual franchisees' failures to comply with wage and hour laws, and pay their workers properly. However, a 2014 ruling by the National Labor Relations Act made all corporations liable for the labor conditions of their franchise operations.[50,51] In light of its huge number of franchisees, this ruling is likely to impact no one more severely than Subway.

Not surprisingly, Subway was a chosen target of the fast food worker strikes demanding higher wages and a union organized by SEIU in 2013 and 2014. In some cases, the company allegedly retaliated against workers who participated in these strikes. In New Jersey in 2014, Subway "sandwich artists" voted to unionize one of their restaurants. The workers worked at a Pilot Flying J's, a travel center that bills itself as Subway's largest nontraditional franchisee. The company ran antiunion meetings to kill the process, but the workers voted in the union despite these efforts.[52] In Seattle, Washington, Subway "sandwich artist'" Carlos Hernandez was supported by Good Jobs Seattle in filing a federal lawsuit against the national Subway corporation alleging wrongful termination and illegal retaliation for striking in 2013.[53] Hernandez was officially fired for giving away a cookie to a child, but he believes he was terminated for trying to organize his coworkers to take part in strikes.[54]

Perhaps these challenges can be passed off as the cost of rapid growth. In an interview with inc.com, Fred de Luca indicated that the company's growth was reliant on supporting franchisees. As mentioned earlier, Subway created a unique program that elevated and paid successful franchisees to train and support an even wider network of franchises.[55] Yet even franchisees, the group that Subway seems to care the most about, have had issues with the rapid growth model. Subway franchisees have complained of feeling exploited by Doctor's Associates Inc., Subway's franchising operation, and being threatened with losing their stores.[56,57] The Federal

Trade Commission has disclosed over 160 legal disputes between Subway and franchisees. U.S. House of Representatives staff economist Dean Sagar said, "Subway is the biggest problem in franchising and emerges as one of the key examples of every abuse you can think of." In one case, the U.S. Small Business Administration challenged a contract clause between Subway and its franchises that gave the international corporation the right to seize and purchase any franchise without cause. The SBA refused small business loans to Subway franchise owners until Subway removed the clause. Franchisees also complain that new Subway stores open close to theirs and create local competition, high royalty costs, and rapid eviction during disputes.[58]

The most-high-profile dispute between Subway and its franchises involved Lt. Col. Leon Batie Jr., who owned two Subway stores in Dallas, Texas. Batie had been deployed to Afghanistan in March 2005, three years after buying his first restaurant. While Batie was deployed by the military in Afghanistan, his stores fell behind on rent. The Subway Real Estate Corp. seized Batie's stores and sold them to a local developer, who resold one of the properties for a $100,000 profit. Batie charged the Subway Corporation with violating the Servicemembers Civil Relief Act by terminating an active duty member's lease without a court order. Subway settled the case; Batie had sought over $5 million in damages in his action.[59–60]

Sandy's Story

Sandy is a native of Detroit, Michigan. After getting married and having a daughter, Sandy started working part time at Subway in 1995, just a few years after the company started franchising stores in Michigan. She started working as a sandwich artist, prepping vegetables, making sandwiches, working the cash register, and cleaning up. Her daughter was 5 years old, and although it wasn't absolutely necessary to work, Sandy wanted the extra income. "I was earning more or less the minimum wage. I was married at that time. I had a husband who had a good job. Most of the other workers there also had families to support, but no other income. Most other people at Subway were on food stamps."

Sandy's situation changed when she got a divorce. She moved to working full time, still for just about $7 an hour. Fortunately, her ex-husband provided child support. "Without the child support, I would have had to go on food stamps."

Sandy ended up working at Subway for sixteen years, from the age of 29 to the age of 45. She remained with the company through a number of franchisee ownership shifts and changes, and ultimately rose to manager. Even in a managerial role, she earned a mere $9 per hour. She remained dependent on child support to live.

Sandy reported extremely high turnover at Subway—and not just of the workers. "I worked in over twenty Subway restaurants. There were hundreds of people who worked there while I was there—there was really high turnover. At least half of these people were older adults working to support families, who had no other income except Subway." The regular turnover of franchise owners creates a culture of impermanence in which employees are regularly moved or let go *en masse*. But Sandy also worked for many different franchise owners. "I was constantly asked to move to a new restaurant to open a new store of the franchisee. Some owners who we worked for, they ended up selling, they didn't want to hire any of us. We had to go to a different Subway."

The transience inherent to Subway's franchise structure led to Sandy's departure from the company. "The last Subway I worked at, a guy walked in and said he was the new owner. We hadn't been told anything. He just came into work and told us were all being let go."

Sandy, who now works elsewhere in the restaurant industry, attributes the instability of working at Subway to the instability of Subway's franchise owners. This results in dramatic swings in workplace treatment and available hours.

What makes Subway franchises different from other franchises is its low barrier to entry for investors. "It takes $10,000 to open up a Subway; it's a lot more to open up a McDonald's. That's why you see Subways everywhere. Anybody can open one up. It's mostly small business folks who don't know anything about restaurants. They'll try to start you for lower than $6 an hour. They think they can treat you any kind of way."

THE HIGH ROAD: ZINGERMAN'S: VISION BEFORE GROWTH

Paul Saginaw was born in Detroit in 1951. Saginaw grew up in a Jewish household in a racially integrated neighborhood of Detroit, where he attended a racially integrated school. Saginaw's family lived within the city of Detroit until 1965, when his parents, like many in that era, left urban areas in favor of new suburban developments—the movement patterns historically known as white flight. "My father tells the story: I had come from school and gotten an A on a paper that had grammatical and spelling errors. My dad thought, 'the schools aren't any good anymore,' and that's when we left."

Trouble found Saginaw for the first time when he left the city. "I never experienced any trouble until we moved to the suburbs. We moved into a subdivision that was mostly Jewish, but next door was a subdivision that wasn't, and we'd take the same bus. The very first week there, I was called a kike. That had never happened back in the 'hood." Saginaw's best friends remained the ones he'd made living in the city.

Saginaw grew up in close proximity to his two grandfathers, and both had a formative impact on his life. He describes one of the grandfathers as "a laborer, a house painter who was very proud of his physique." The other grandfather, a man named Ben Sherman, owned a small business that focused on reconditioning and reselling used ball bearings. Saginaw remembers his grandfather Sherman for his generosity. Sherman, a European Jewish immigrant, posed as a cousin to other immigrants who wished to move to the United States, thereby smoothing their immigration process. "We grew up with people around us who weren't really related," Saginaw recalls. "[Sherman] was extremely generous. He always told me, 'Half of what you have belongs to those who need it.' It meant that if you become successful, you have to make the people around you successful.

"You don't shit on the rungs as you climb the ladder of success, because they're the same ones you'll come down on the way down."

Learning about Giving

Saginaw would go to work with his grandfather and watch how he operated. His grandfather's ball bearing shop was at Six Mile, then a rough neighborhood of Detroit. People would come into the shop asking for money, and Saginaw's grandfather always responded the same way. "There was a bar next door that served hamburgers. Grandpa would say, 'Go next door, have a meal, tell them to put it on Mr. Sherman's tab.' Everything he said built up over time. I don't know if anyone influenced the way I live and think in the world more than my grandfather."

Men in Saginaw's family each espoused an appreciation for having comfort while stopping short of excess. "I grew up where no one was trying to get wealthy. There is such a thing as enough. People were focused on taking care of other people. It was not a mindset of scarcity, but a spirit of generosity. People lived a modest lifestyle, and they were not worried about losing their roof or where their next meal was going to come from."

Drawn from this outlook was an appreciation for work, which Saginaw relates in a story about a bike he wanted when he was 14. "It was $199.95. I told my dad, 'I want you to buy this for me,' and he said, 'Go earn your own money.'" Saginaw found a landscaping job after school. Fridays he'd get an envelope with cash in it. "It was such a wonderful feeling. Since that day, I've never been without a job. Just the act of working was such a wonderful feeling of satisfaction, pride; I loved it."

Finding the Path

A self-described "terrible student" who "barely got out of high school," Saginaw bounced around between jobs and college intermittently over a span of nine years. "I had basic intelligence, I just wasn't a good classroom learner." Ultimately he emerged with a degree in zoology from the University of Michigan.

While in Ann Arbor, Saginaw found an additional interest in another subject: his roommate, Lori. Lori was a Japanese-American daughter of a Baptist minister and a recent graduate of Kalamazoo College—"the Harvard of the Midwest," as Saginaw describes it—who was living in Ann Arbor to pursue a teaching certificate. She also had a boyfriend. "I told my friends, 'I met this girl and I'm going to marry her.'" Saginaw succeeded in his quest to marry Lori. "Our families were both against it—she wasn't Jewish, she wasn't white. My sisters came to the wedding but no one else from my family. My grandmother had forbidden everyone to come. Many years later, my mother believed she was at my wedding (in her mind). I always kept the door open; it was their loss. When my grandma died, that allowed my mother to normalize things. Now my father is going to be 96, and my wife spends a lot of time taking care of him."

Entering the Industry

After getting married, Saginaw took jobs at restaurants in Ann Arbor. He started as a bartender. "I didn't know how to make drinks but [the owner] thought I had a good personality. I made flashcards and learned all the drinks overnight."

After Saginaw quickly rose from bartender to bar manager and kitchen manager, he was asked by the owner to become General Manager of a second restaurant down the block. It was there that he met Ari Weinzweig, a Chicago native who had recently graduated from the University of Michigan with a degree in Russian history, specializing in anarchists. "He wanted to get a job as a waiter, but we didn't have an opening, so he washed dishes."

Saginaw and Weinzweig quickly became very close, bonding over their shared nostalgia for the neighborhood delicatessens of their hometowns. "Ann Arbor was a wasteland for stuff like that," Saginaw recalls. "We thought that could be a good business. At one point there was a grocery store across the street from our restaurant that was sold to a new landlord. The new owner knew I had managed restaurants, and asked if I'd like to be partners with him to open the restaurant. I said no but that I'd like to lease the space from him to open my own."

A Unique Vision of Growth

Early one Sunday morning, Saginaw went to Weinzweig's house to wake him and tell him about the location for their new business. They sat down at a Smith Corona typewriter and started to write out a business plan and vision. "Our idea was to gather the finest products and have a specialty food store. We envisioned a busy bustling sandwich shop with overstuffed corned beef sandwiches." Even in these early days they set out a shared vision for how they would grow their business: slowly. "We said we wanted it to be unique and extraordinary, that it could never be replicated if it grew. I've never seen an operation that expanded [quickly] that got better."

The two owners thought about employee wages and benefits, too. "The way I thought about it from the very beginning was I wanted a business that was a vehicle for positive social change. The truth is that if you're in business and you're not responsible, you're putting a lot of people at risk. To me, the purpose of business was not the creation of wealth for shareholders. It was to give everyone connected with it a better life. That was the lesson I had learned from my grandfather—you have this obligation to share success."

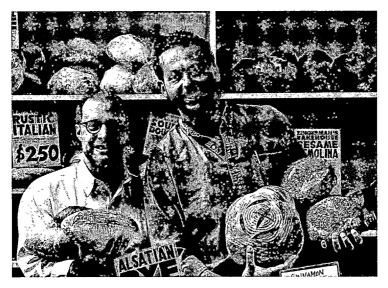

Paul Saginaw and Ari Weinzweig.

Part of Saginaw's vision was a belief that every worker could be involved in the steering and creation of the company's vision. "We wanted a strategy that sought to promote this human potential that surrounds us. We're in a business where everyone has some of the ingredients that are necessary to be successful [and] we can encourage them to take action. That's what we wanted to do with it."

Saginaw and Weinzweig were also committed to the same standard of human potential discovery among suppliers. "We wanted to support people to make great food. From the day we opened, we were always looking for tiny producers. Others would say to us, 'Why don't you cut down [the] number of suppliers?'" Convenience was not the criteria; quality and community were.

Over time, Saginaw and Weinzweig have expanded—and diversified. The Zingerman's Community of Businesses (ZCoB) is the company's portfolio of specialized operations, one that embodies their commitment to slow, sustainable growth. The ZCoB encompasses ten businesses: the original Zingerman's Delicatessen, Zingerman's Bakehouse, Zingerman's Catering and Events, Zingerman's Mail Order, Zingerman's Creamery, Zingerman's Roadhouse, Zingerman's Coffee, Zingerman's Candy Factory, Zingerman's Cornman Farms, and ZingTrain—a consulting and training firm that teaches other companies how to build in the Zingerman's way. Totaling more than 600 employees, the network of businesses complement each other without redundancy, creating an ecosystem of food, services, and employment; it is the antithesis of a franchising model. "We wanted to be unique, so that if you were craving a Zingerman's sandwich, you'd have to come all the way to Ann Arbor. The longer we've been at it, the more fun it has become. We certainly have watched many of our colleagues sell out, take the money and run. But we didn't. It wouldn't have been any fun."

Although each Zingerman's business in unique, all come together in a joint partnership model that maintains quality standards for both products and employment. "We're not Subway sandwiches—we use real food. Most things are made in house. We're concerned about the integrity of the product, how it's grown, processed, and packaged. Some people say, 'Of course your prices are high—you're paying more.' No. The cost of food is determined by the cost of ingredients."

Although Zingerman's price points are higher than those of a restaurant like Subway, their sandwich prices are by no means exorbitant. Many Zingerman's sandwiches cost $10—or just $2 more than some footlong sandwiches at Subway. On the topic of prices, Saginaw is careful to note that the difference between Zingerman's and their competitors is not just price. "That price isn't just the cost of a sandwich; it's the cost of a wonderful meal. How many times have you gone to a fine dining restaurant and it's $25 and you're sorely disappointed?"

Taking the High Road

Zingerman's strives to offer wages and benefits far above the minimum: their minimum entry-level wage is currently $9, and will increase to $11 by January 2016. Many workers start higher than that, and after orientation wages go up again. Workers are entitled to one week of paid personal time off (including sick leave and vacation), increasing to two weeks after two years and three weeks after three years.

Tipped workers at Zingerman's Roadhouse, the company's only full-service restaurant, earn $2.77, which is the minimum legal wage for tipped workers in Michigan. Saginaw says the company is moving to change that to the full minimum wage. With their newest Zingerman's restaurant, a Korean restaurant, the company has decided to move to no tips and instead provide servers with a livable wage. "I don't want the people who are working for us to be struggling. It's embarrassing that we're asking people to prepare this wonderful food, give great service, if they can't go home and give great service to their children. In our [year] 2020 vision, we say that we want the financial success that's experienced by the business to be mirrored in our staff." Saginaw's method: "We need training in personal finance, budgeting, even how to buy a house. We want to get them on firm, more stable financial ground."

"We should not be asking the customer to decide whether our worker gets a livable wage."

The final frontier for ZCoB is employee ownership. The organization is structured such that Zingerman's employees can propose and receive financing to start a new business within the ZCoB. "If you're passionate and operate according to our guiding principles, we would finance you, and that's how we created the community of businesses. It's a clear, transparent process."

The Zingerman's ownership team is cognizant that not all 600 employees are going to open their own Zingerman's business. The question, then, became how to structure ownership—or at least ownership empowerment—among employees who don't helm their own Zingerman's imprint. At first, Saginaw pioneered the concept of open-book management: training all workers in the company finances, price setting, and management so that everyone had the opportunity to weigh in on the company's business practices. Then, in 2010, Saginaw attended a conference of the Business Alliance for Local Living Economies (BALLE), where he saw a presentation on the history of corporations. Saginaw recalls hearing the presenter say, "the traditional corporation is the last plantation" and feeling gutted. "That was like an arrow to my heart. I thought, 'is that true?' It prodded me to want to spread ownership deeper and wider in the organization." As a result, Zingerman's started offering employee ownership to workers throughout the company, and inducted its first worker members onto the partnership board of ZCoB.

"I think we've always thought we were going to measure our success not by what we were gaining but by what we were contributing to our coworkers and our community. We wanted to operate with a mentality of abundance and a spirit of generosity. There's a natural progression toward wider ownership. Now we've reached a point where we can start to share ownership and control more widely."

NOTES

1. Subway: Explore Our World, http://www.subway.com/subwayroot/exploreourworld.aspx (accessed 23 February 2015).
2. "The History of Subway," *Subway*, http://www.subway.com/subwayroot/about_us/history.aspx (accessed 2 July, 2015).
3. Scott Eason, "Making Billions Ain't Rocket Science!," CNBC, November 5, 2007, <http://www.cnbc.com/id/21636472>
4. Burt Helm, "The Sandwich That Ate the World," *Inc.com*, April 30, 2013. <http://www.inc.com/magazine/201305/burt-helm/how-i-did-it-fred-deluca-subway.html>
5. Ibid.
6. "Subway: Explore Our World," *Subway*, http://www.subway.com/subwayroot/exploreourworld.aspx (accessed July 2, 2015); "What It Is like to Work at Subway." *Indeed.com*, http://www.indeed.com/cmp/Subway?from=reviews (accessed 23 February 2015).
7. Karlene Lukovitz, "New Subway Campaign Spotlights Veggies," *Media Post*, August 4, 2014. http://www.mediapost.com/publications/article/231264/new-subway-campaign-spotlights-veggies.html.
8. Eric Schroeder, "Subway recognizes suppliers for improving bread," *Baking Business*, January 22, 2015. http://www.bakingbusiness.com/articles/news_home/Food-Service/2015/01/Subway_recognizes_suppliers_fo.aspx?ID=%7BBE7821B6-5E46-4593-823E-C7A64B4F7FE7%7D&cck=1.
9. "Jared Fogle's career as Subway spokesman after losing 245 pounds," *Washington Post*, July 8, 2015, http://www.washingtonpost.com/lifestyle/style/jared-fogle/2015/07/08/b351479c-2560-11e5-aae2-6c4f59b050aa_gallery.html.
10. Rheana Murray, , "Subway commercial spokesman Jared Fogle marks 15 years of turkey subs and keeping the weight off," *NY Daily News*, June 9, 2013, http://www.nydailynews.com/life-style/health/jared-subway-guy-marks-15-years-turkey-subs-article-1.1365511.

11. Jared Fogle, and Anthony Bruno, *Jared, the Subway Guy: Winning Through Losing: 13 Lessons for Turning Your Life Around* (New York, NY: St. Martin's Press,.2006), 82.

12. Ben Forer, "Subway Cuts Salt in 'Fresh Fit' sandwiches," ABC News, April 18, 2011, http://abcnews.go.com/Health/subway-cuts-salt-fresh-fit-sandwiches/story?id=13399837.

13. Rohan Dua, "Subway to Roll Out World's 1st All-Veg Outlet in Punjab," *India Times*, August 17, 2012, http://timesofindia.indiatimes.com/city/chandigarh/Subway-to-roll-out-worlds-1st-all-veg-outlet-in-Punjab/articleshow/15526098.cms?referral=PM; "Get Your Vegan On!," *We Love Subway*, accessed July 2, 2015. http://welovesubway.com/.

14. Bridget Albert, "Subway Restaurant Committed to Proper Treatment of Animals," *New Haven Register,* September 15, 2012, http://www.nhregister.com/general-news/20120915/subway-restaurants-committed-to-proper-treatment-of-animals. However, as of the date of that article, only 4 percent of the eggs served by Subway in the US and Canada were free range.

15. "Environmental Leadership," *Subway,* http://www.subway.com/subwayroot/about_us/Social_Responsibility/EnvironmentalLeadership.aspx (accessed July 9 2015).

16. Alicia Kelso, "Subway Continues Commitment to Eco Restaurant Model," QSR Web, October 18, 2011. http://www.qsrweb.com/articles/subway-continues-commitment-to-eco-restaurant-model/.

17. Rachel Tepper, "McDonald's and Subway Nutrition Can Be Equally Bad for Teens, Study Finds," *Huffington Post*, May 9, 2013, http://www.huffingtonpost.com/2013/05/09/mcdonalds-subway-nutrition-teens_n_3246268.html.

18. Nanci Hellmich. "Subway's 'Health Halo' Can Lead People to Consume More Calories," *USA Today*, September 30, 2007, http://usatoday30.usatoday.com/news/health/2007-09-30-mcsubway_N.htm.

19. Anne Shooter, "Invasion of the Super-Sized Sarnies: As Subway Overtakes McDonalds as Our Biggest Fast-Food Chain, the Artery Clogging Truth About Its Sandwiches." *Daily Mail*, March 11, 2011. < http://www.dailymail.co.uk/health/article-1365424/Subway-vs-McDonalds-The-artery-clogging-truth-favourite-fast-food-chains.html>

20. Hayley Peterson, "Former Subway Operator Threatens to Leak '$35 Million' in Sandwich Secrets." *Business Insider,* Aug. 7, 2014. <http://www.businessinsider.com/subway-owner-threatens-sandwich-secrets-2014-8>; Polly Mosendz, "There's A Man Trying to Blackmail Subway with Sandwich Secrets Worth $35 Million." *The Wire,* Aug. 6, 2014. <http://www.thewire.com/business/2014/08/there-is-a-man-trying-to-blackmail-subway-with-sandwich-secrets-worth-35-million/375698/>.

21. Chris Vedelago, "Subway 'Secrets' Revealed as Alleged Blackmailer Takes on 'Sandwich Mafia.'" *The Age*, August 6, 2014. <http://www.theage.com.au/victoria/subway-secrets-revealed-as-alleged-blackmailer-takes-on-sandwich-mafia-20140806-100swe.html>.

22. "Subway Secret Recipe to Deceive the Customers Revealed," August 4, 2014, Online video clip, Youtube.com, https://www.youtube.com/watch?v=Sn_8l5r24GA#t=43 (accessed March 28, 2014).

23. Justin Andress,. "Video Allegedly Posted by Ex-Subway Franchisee Shows Misleading 'Health' Tactics." *Examiner*, Aug. 6, 2014, <http://www.examiner.com/article/video-allegedly-posted-by-ex-subway-franchisee-shows-misleading-health-tactics>

24. Tracy Miller, "Subway Will Remove Additive Found in Plastics from Its Bread After Blogger's Online Petition," *NewYork Daily News*, February 6, 2014, http://www.nydailynews.com/life-style/health/subway-remove-additive-found-plastics-bread-article-1.1604610.

25. Bruce Horovitz, "Subway to Remove Chemical from Bread," *USA Today*, February 10, 2014.

26. "Subway: No More 'Yoga Mat' Chemical in our Bread," CBS News, April 14, 2014, http://www.cbsnews.com/news/subway-no-more-yoga-mat-chemical-in-our-bread/.

27. Elizabeth Landau, "Subway to Remove 'Dough Conditioner' Chemical from Bread," CNN, February 17, 2014, http://www.cnn.com/2014/02/06/health/subway-bread-chemical/.

28. "List of Substances That Can Cause Occupational Asthma," Health and Safety Executive, United Kingdom <http://www.hse.gov.uk/asthma/substances.htm> (accessed July 2, 2015).

29. Melanie Warner, "At Subway, Customers Really Aren't Eating as 'Fresh' as They Think," CBS News, April 18, 2011, http://www.cbsnews.com/news/at-subway-customers-really-arent-eating-as-fresh-as-they-think/.

30. Ryan Hoffman, "Norovirus Outbreak in BV Serves as Warning," *The Mountain Mail*, December 9, 2014. <http://www.themountainmail.com/free_content/article_27b20560-7fba-11e4-8e28-574b8e79feba.html>

31. Reuven Blau. "Subway Restaurants Have Been Closed for Health Violations More Than Any Other Chain in the City," *New York Daily News*, April 18, 2012, http://www.nydailynews.com/new-york/subway-restaurants-closed-health-violations-chain-city-article-1.1063271.

32. Ibid.

33. Aina Hunter, "Subway Salmonella Scare: Woman Sues Restaurant Chain After Outbreak Sickens 97 in Illinois," *CBS News*, June 23, 2010, http://www.cbsnews.com/news/subway-salmonella-scare-woman-sues-restaurant-chain-after-outbreak-sickens-97-in-illinois/.

34. Zach Mallove, "Lawsuits Filed in Subway Shigella Outbreak," *Food Safety News*, March 12, 2010, http://www.foodsafetynews.com/2010/03/two-lawsuits-filed-in-subway-oubtreak.

35. Chris Morran, "Chicago-Area Subway Now Being Blamed for 78 Illnesses," *Consumerist*, March 18, 2010. http://consumerist.com/2010/03/18/chicago-area-subway-now-being-blamed-for-78-illnesses/.

36. ROC United, "Behind the Kitchen Door: A Multi-Site Study of the Restaurant Industry," February 14, 2011. <http://rocunited.org/2011-behind-the-kitchen-door-multi-site-study/>

37. Mary Bottari, "The 'Other NRA,' the National Restaurant Association, Pushes Preemption of Paid Sick Days," *PR Watch*, Center for Media and Democracy, July 24, 2014, http://www.prwatch.org/news/2013/07/12173/other-nra-national-restaurant-association-pushes-preemption-paid-sick-days>; "Opposition to Paid Sick Days," *Source Watch*, Center for Media and Democracy, http://www.sourcewatch.org/index.php/National_Restaurant_Association#Opposition_to_Paid_Sick_Days(accessed July 7, 2015).

38. Emily Thomas, "Subway Worker Claims She Was Forced to Work While Vomiting," *Huffington Post*, July 17, 2014, http://www.huffingtonpost.com/2014/07/17/sick-subway-worker-elizabeth-taff_n_5593377.html. In an "Update" to its article, the *Huffington Post* reported that it had received a statement from Subway in which the Freeport, Texas franchisee claimed that the worker's "allegations are not true."

39. C. A. Pinkman, "Subway Forces Violently Sick Employee to Keep Working, Then Fires Her." *Jezebel*, July 16, 2014. < http://kitchenette.jezebel.com/subway-forces-violently-ill-employee-to-keep-working-t-1606340974?utm_campaign=socialflow_jezebel_facebook&utm_source=jezebel_facebook&utm_medium=socialflow>; Syan Rhodes, "Subway Worker Says She Was Forced to Serve Food to Customers While Sick." < http://www.click2houston.com/news/subway-worker-says-she-was-forced-to-serve-food-to-customers-while-sick/26978808>.

40. "Workers' Access to Paid Sick Days in the States," Institute for Women's Policy Research and National Partnership for Women and Families, May 2015. http://www.nationalpartnership.org/research-library/work-family/psd/workers-access-to-paid-sick-days-in-the-states.pdf>; "Current Paid Sick Days Laws," National Partnership for Women and Families, June 26, 2015. <http://www.nationalpartnership.org/research-library/work-family/psd/current-paid-sick-days-laws.pdf>

41. "Fact Sheet: White House Unveils New Steps to Strengthen Working Families Across America," Office of the Press Secretary, The White House, January 14, 2015. < https://www.whitehouse.gov/the-press-office/2015/01/14/fact-sheet-white-house-unveils-new-steps-strengthen-working-families-acr>.

42. "Job Descriptions: Sandwich Artist," <https://www.mysubwaycareer.com/Home/JobDescriptions?clt=en-US>(accessed July 9, 2015).

43. "Super-Sizing Public Costs: How Low Wages at Top Fast-Food Chains Leave Taxpayers Footing the Bill," Data Brief, National Employment Law Project, October 2013. p. 2. http://www.nelp.org/content/uploads/2015/03/NELP-Super-Sizing-Public-Costs-Fast-Food-Report.pdf.

44. Annalyn Kurtz, "Subway Leads Fast Food Industry in Underpaying Workers." *CNN Money*, May 1, 2014, http://money.cnn.com/2014/05/01/news/economy/subway-labor-violations/.

45. Annalyn Kurtz, "Subway CEO: 'No Excuse' for Wage Violations." *CNN Money*, May 9, 2014, <http://money.cnn.com/2014/05/09/news/economy/subway-ceo-wage-violations/>

46. "Subway Franchise Owner in Buffalo, Minnesota, to Pay 16 Workers Back Wages, Damages After US Labor Department Investigation Finds Falsified Time Records." News Release, Department of Labor, September 17, 2014, <http://www.dol.gov/opa/media/press/whd/WHD20141600.htm>.

47. "US Labor Department sues Subway Franchisee to Recover Back Wages, Damages for 68 Employees of 5 Ohio Eateries." News Release, Department of Labor, February 6, 2012, http://www.dol.gov/whd/media/press/whdpressVB3.asp?pressdoc=Midwest/20120206.xml.

48. "US Labor Department's Wage and Hour Division and SUBWAY Franchisor Collaborate to Boost Restaurants' Compliance with Federal Labor Laws." News Release, Department of Labor. May 8, 2013. http://www.dol.gov/opa/media/press/whd/WHD20130687.htm.

49. Katie Little, "Subway CEO: How I'd Solve the Minimum Wage Debate." *CNBC*, May 7, 2014.

50. Susan Adams, "McDonald's Loses Big Labor Ruling," *Forbes*, July 30, 2014, http://www.forbes.com/sites/susanadams/2014/07/30/mcdonalds-loses-big-labor-ruling.

51. Michael J. Lotitio, and Missy Parry, "A New 'Fact Sheet' for Franchises at the NLRB," *Franchising World*, March 16, 2015. http://franchisingworld.com/a-new-fact-sheet-for-franchises-at-the-nlrb/.

52. Dave Jamieson, "Workers at a Subway sandwich shop vote to unionize," *Huffington Post*, July 21, 2014, http://www.huffingtonpost.com/2014/07/21/subway-union-election-rwdsu_n_5607006.html.

53. Angela Nickerson, "Labor Rights Group Sues Subway for Firing Striker," *The Capitol Hill Times*, October 3, 2013, http://www.capitolhilltimes.com/2013/10/labor-rights-group-sues-subway-firing-striker.

54. Ashley Gross, "Fast Food Worker Challenges Firing, But Faces Uphill Battle," KPLU 88.5, September 24, 2013, http://kplu.org/post/fast-food-worker-challenges-firing-faces-uphill-battle.

55. Burt Helm, "The Sandwich That Ate the World," Inc.com, April 30, 2013. <http://www.inc.com/magazine/201305/burt-helm/how-i-did-it-fred-deluca-subway.html>.
56. "Subway Franchise Horror Stories: How Not to Become One," Unhappy Franchisee, October 10, 2012, http://www.unhappyfranchisee.com/category/franchisor/subway-franchisor/ (accessed 24 February 2015).
57. Susan Berfield, "Jared Isn't Subway's Only Problem: Dark Times for the World's Biggest Fast Food Chain," *Bloomberg Business*, July 9, 2015, http://www.bloomberg.com/news/features/2015-07-09/jared-isn-t-subway-s-only-problem.
58. Richard Behar, "Why SubwayIis 'the Biggest Problem in Franchising' That's the Assessment of a Congressional Staffer Who Studied the Industry. Founder Fred DeLuca's Unique Approach to the Sandwich Business has Brought Him Staggering Wealth—and Big Troubles," *Fortune*, March 16, 1998, http://archive.fortune.com/magazines/fortune/fortune_archive/1998/03/16/239302/index.htm.
59. Karen Robinson-Jacobs, "Subway, Soldier Settle Dallas Franchise Dispute," *Dallas News*, January 4, 2010, http://www.dallasnews.com/business/headlines/20100104-Subway-soldier-settle-Dallas-franchise-3530.ece.
60. *Batie v. Subway Real Estate Corp.,* No. 3:07-CV-1415-M, 2008 (N.D. Tex. Feb. 15, 2008). http://www.gpo.gov/fdsys/pkg/USCOURTS-txnd-3_07-cv-01415/pdf/USCOURTS-txnd-3_07-cv-01415-0.pdf.

[7]

THE COFFEE CAFÉ

Place for Debate?

The earliest recorded coffee houses were controversial as a gathering place for discussion, debate, and dissent. Some of the earliest coffee houses were found in the Ottoman Empire of the sixteenth century, in which imams feared and banned the coffee house as a place that took people away from the Mosque and where dissent was fomented.[1] Coffee finally came to Europe from the Ottoman Empire in the seventeenth century. As in Cairo and Damascus, coffee houses in London grew quickly and became places for debate and discussion. Like Ottoman rulers, King Charles II feared coffee houses in London as gathering places for dissenters against the King. Men (and only men) of all social classes gathered to criticize the government and debate news and political events.[2] French coffee houses emerged slightly later in the same century and became major meeting places for the dissent of the greatest French philosophers and thinkers, along with disaffected bourgeoisie, which may even have been a factor that led to the French Revolution.[3]

In 1950s and 1960s America, coffee houses also became a place for political conversation and political music, particularly folk music.[4] And although Seattle became known for its coffee houses, locations of debate and dissent, the most famous of Seattle-based coffee houses, Starbucks, can hardly be called a hotbed of political conversation. Far from being a gathering place for conversation and dissent, even Starbucks workers attempting to speak up to improve the company's working conditions and low wages have faced retaliation on the job.[5-6] Fortunately, there are a number of coffee shops and cafes in America who think very differently about room for dissent. See Tables 7.1 and 7.2.

THE LOW ROAD: STARBUCKS

Jerry Baldwin, Zev Siegel, and Gordon Bowker were students at the University of San Francisco with a shared adoration of Peet's Coffee and Tea, a Berkeley, California, coffee-roasting company founded by Dutch immigrant Alfred Peet.[7]

Eager to replicate Peet's model of importing and roasting exceptional coffee, they founded their own coffee company using individual buy-ins of $1,350 and a collective loan of $5,000 borrowed from the bank.[8,9]

The three partners opened their business in 1971 in Seattle's Pike Place Market. They called the store Starbucks, after the character in *Moby Dick*, to evoke "the romance of the high seas and the seafaring tradition of the early coffee traders."[10] Their logo featured a twin-tailed siren from Greek Mythology.[11] For the first year of operation, Starbucks purchased coffee beans from Peet's Coffee. Soon after, Starbucks set up its own roasting operations.[12]

Sales exceeded expectations for the first store, and a second location was opened in Seattle after one year. Incremental growth continued through the company's first decade. Zev Siegel, one of the founders, left the company in the early 1980s, leaving Bowker and Baldwin as owners and operators of four Seattle locations.[13,14]

Table 7.1 LOW-ROAD RESTAURANTS

	$10+ Wage for Non-Tipped Workers	Hourly Wage for Tipped Workers Exceeds Minimum	Paid Sick Days	Promotion Practices	Stars
Au Bon Pain		n/a*			
Bruegger's Bagel Bakery					
Caribou Coffee					
Dunkin' Donuts		n/a*			
Einstein Bros. Bagels		n/a*			
La Madeleine Country French Cafe		n/a*			
Panera		n/a*		←	
Starbucks					
Tim Horton's		n/a*			

*No tipped employees.

Table 7.2 HIGH-ROAD RESTAURANTS

	$10+ Wage for Non-Tipped Workers	Hourly Wage for Tipped Workers Exceeds Minimum	Paid Sick Days	Promotion Practices	Stars
3 Worlds Café Los Angeles, CA	💵	💲+		←	★★★
Arizmendi San Francisco, CA	💵	💲+		n/a	★
Cafe Gabriela Oakland, CA	💵	💲+		←	★★★
Choices Vegan Café Miami, FL	💵	💲+		←	★★★
Haley House Bakery Café Boston, MA	💵	n/a*		←	★
Manifesto Café Los Angeles, CA		💲+	▬●	n/a	★

Pacha Organic Café *Austin, TX*	💵	💲+		←	★★
Peet's Coffee and Tea *National*	💵			←	★
Pleasant Pops *Washington, DC*	💵	n/a*	🌡	←	★★
The Random Tea Room & Curiosity Shop *Philadelphia, PA*	n/a	💲+		←	★

*No tipped employees.

In 1981, Howard Schultz—then a vice president and general manager for a Swedish kitchen equipment company called Hammarplast—walked into a Starbucks location and found himself taken by the store's flavorful coffee. His interest in the company was so great that he asked for (and was granted) a meeting with Bowker and Baldwin, where he praised the owners for their focus on maximizing the quality of the coffee and educating customers about the different qualities of fine coffees.[15,16]

Schultz asked to work for Starbucks; the co-founders were not entirely sure. They worried about hiring an outsider with a very different outlook on business development, one who could potentially want to take the company in a very different direction. Schultz persisted for nearly a year. Eventually, they hired him in 1982 as director of retail operations and marketing.[17] This led to a period of rapid growth for Starbucks, one that was accelerated in 1987 when Schultz led a group that purchased the company from its founders. Years later, when asked a question about Schultz, Gordon Bowker responded: "If you can't say something nice about somebody, don't say anything at all."[18]

Under Schultz's leadership, Starbucks grew into an empire, with more than 21,000 stores in 65 countries[19] and 191,000 employees.[20] In 2008, Starbucks announced its "transformation agenda," a set of business and development goals that extended into other social and industrial arenas as well: "(1) Be the undisputed coffee authority; (2) engage and inspire staff [also known as 'Partners']; (3) ignite the emotional attachment to customers; (4) expand global presence while making each store the heart of the local neighborhood; (5) be the leader in ethical sourcing and environmental impact; (6) creative innovative growth platforms worthy of Starbuck's coffee; (7) deliver a sustainable economic model."[21]

Publicizing the High Road

Starbucks has gone to great lengths to publicize their employment practices, which they claim are above industry standards. Referring to line-level workers as "partners," Starbucks proudly claims: "We believe in treating our partners with respect and dignity. We are proud to offer two landmark programs for our partners: comprehensive health coverage for eligible full- and part-time partners and equity in the company through *Bean Stock*."[22] In 1988, Starbucks began offering full health benefits to eligible full and part-time employees.[23] In 1991, Starbucks became the first privately owned U.S. company to offer a stock option program that includes part-time employees.[24] The company proclaims that employees get to take home a pound of coffee each week and get a 30 percent discount on food and beverages.[25]

In 2014, the company announced the "Starbucks College Achievement Plan to help thousands of U.S. Starbucks partners (employees) complete their education."[26] This free college tuition plan is offered to full time and part-time employees and allows them to take online classes at Arizona State University. Starbucks also provides an "enrollment coach, financial aid counselor, and academic advisor to support them through graduation."[27] In publicizing the program, Howard Shultz, CEO of Starbucks proclaimed, "There's no doubt, the inequality within the country has created a situation where many Americans are being left behind. Everyone who works as hard as our partners do should have the opportunity to complete college, while balancing work, school and their personal lives."[28]

Unfortunately, not all Starbucks "partners" agree with that Starbucks is doing all that it should for its workers. Over the last several years, a group of Starbucks workers formed the Starbucks Workers Union (SWU), which claims that "Across the world, Starbucks pays its 100% part-time barista workforce poverty wages, and busts unions when [workers "come together" for change, even while raking in over $1.7 billion in profits this year."[29,30] Workers complain about understaffed stores, but Starbucks denies the understaffing claims.[31] A study by the Starbucks Workers Union found that Starbucks staffs its stores with "about 16 workers per stores, compared to almost 19 before the recession."[32] Interviews with Starbucks employees found that, "Even those who say they like their job paint a picture of a business that underpays front-line workers, enforces work rules arbitrarily, and too often fails to strike a balance between corporate goals and employee needs."[33] On the whole, the *New York Times* writes, "Starbucks prides itself on progressive labor practices, such as offering health benefits and stock. But its goals—treating workers well and making profits—are in tension. Baristas across the country say that their actual working conditions vary wildly, and that the company often fails to live up to its professed ideals, by refusing to offer any guaranteed hours to part-time workers and keeping many workers' pay at minimum wage."[34]

These complaints could be dismissed as belonging to an isolated group of disgruntled workers who do not represent the majority of Starbucks's massive workforce. However, recent highly publicized controversies indicate that some of these challenges may be more widespread. In August 2014, the *New York Times* reported on Starbucks' "Clopening" practices—having employees scheduled for consecutive closing and opening shifts back to back—in an article titled: "Work Anything but 9 to 5: Scheduling Technology Leaves Low-Income Parents with Hours of Chaos."[35] The article described how "clopening" schedule practices left employees with little to no sleep. Workers were also given little notice of their work schedules, were sent home early if sales were slow, and had extreme variations in hours week to week. These erratic schedules were being set by automated software.[36] Starbucks "drew widespread criticism" after this article appeared,[37] and in response vowed to make schedules more predictable and get rid of "clopening."

Shortly after the *New York Times* article, PBS featured an interview with a Starbucks barista, Liberte Locke, who claims she has suffered repetitive-strain injuries from working 11–12-hour shifts at Starbucks in order to make ends meet. Locke stated that whereas employees are required to give six months' notice of their availability, the automatic online system was only giving employees a week's notice of their schedule. She reported that employees who want to work 32 hours per week have to make themselves available 70 percent of the hours that the store is open; this could be a practical impossibility given that certain stores are only closed three hours per day. Locke reported that a worker needed to be available 100 hours in order to get 32, making it difficult to raise a family, go to school, or have a second job.[38]

In light of this negative publicity, in October 2014 Starbucks announced sweeping changes to employment policies, including tailored individual employee pay raises, increasing starting salaries, providing one free food item to its employees, and allowing workers to display tattoos (except tattoos on the neck or face). The company did not specify the amount by which it would increase salaries.[39] Many attribute this announcement to the controversy Starbucks faced after press reports about the erratic scheduling practices.[40]

Autumn's Story

Autumn grew up alternating residences in Portland, Oregon, where her mother lived, and Seattle, where her father lived. "They were separated when I was really little. But I had a bad relationship with my dad. As a teenager, I had the normal problems with both parents. So I'd go back and forth, trying to figure out the best situation." In her sophomore year of high school, Autumn moved in with her dad in Seattle, and decided to stay.

After high school, Autumn attended South Seattle Community College and worked at Arby's. She took mostly online classes so that she could leave her schedule open to work. Living on her own and paying her own way, her frustrations with working in fast food led her to look elsewhere. In Seattle, Starbucks was a popular counterpoint to traditional fast-food jobs. When Autumn started working at a Starbucks location, she saw the job as a step up. "It was easier than fast food, and people respect the job more." Autumn's hourly wage was $9.50 plus tip shares at Starbucks, an increase from the Washington state minimum wage of $9.39 she made at Arby's.

What Autumn quickly discovered was that work at Starbucks had many of the same trappings as fast-food work. It started with the hours, which were simultaneously inconsistent and scarce. Shifts for Autumn often began at 4:30 A.M. and could be cut short depending on the customer traffic and staff levels. Autumn and her coworkers uniformly struggled to piece together full-time workweeks. "Your schedule really varied week by week—sometimes twenty-five hours, sometimes eighteen hours. Schedules changed every week; I couldn't plan for things a week ahead." Besides making it difficult for Autumn to attend college classes, it also forced her to try to add other (similarly short) shifts at other Starbucks locations.

Starbucks' pay practices made Autumn's struggle for hours even more frustrating. Like many other corporate restaurant chains, Starbucks only offers workers the option of receiving their pay on a debit card or via direct deposit. (Itemized paystubs are accessible only through an inaccessible website that, in Autumn's view, is neither highly visible nor readily accessible.) Autumn first chose to receive the debit card, called a "Global Cash Card," and found it more frustrating than functional. "I kept trying to call their customer service to transfer money from the debit card to my regular bank account, but I could never get a hold of them. You could use the debit card to buy things, but not to pay your rent or bills or anything. You could use it in ATMs but they would charge fees; it was impossible to get cash from your paycheck without paying something."

The scarcity of take-home pay made health insurance and other benefits a non-option for Autumn. "Generally no one had enough hours. If you're only getting 22 hours per week at minimum wage, you have nothing to pay the health insurance. There couldn't have been more than one or two people out of the 10–12 people [working in the Starbucks] who had the health insurance."

The culture and treatment of "partners" at Starbucks made it, in Autumn's experience, actually less livable than working at Arby's. By appearing to be a more desirable alternative to the fast-food job experience, Autumn's Starbucks was an ongoing cycle of quickly disheartened new employees—an extreme version of the high turnover on display in much of the corporate restaurant industry. "A lot of people came looking for a job that was better than fast food—people who had worked at McDonald's. Within the first week I was there, people would just not show up. There were many times when I was not making as much as I used to make at Arby's."

After starting work at Starbucks, Autumn experienced a first in her life: visiting a food bank for groceries.

"I never had to go to a foodbank growing up. It happened for the first time while I was working in Starbucks. The people at the foodbank were nice, but it was kind of embarrassing. When I was at Arby's, I worked there full time, and I could shop at a regular grocery store."

The Starbucks Image

Autumn reports that most Starbucks workers share certain physical traits. "There were some older people supporting kids who were working there, but most people had to fit the image that Starbucks goes for—the young, college educated image. I remember in fast food, everyone had kids, even the younger people. For Starbucks, it seems like they only hire a certain type—younger people who look like they're going to college."

The image also seemed to have a racial component, at least in the particular Starbucks in which Autumn worked, which was in a wealthier residential neighborhood. "It was almost all white people; there were a few Latino workers [who] didn't have accents. They had light skinned tones, and passed as white. While I was there, there was only one African American who ever worked there."

For someone like Autumn—living on her own, going to school, no other income—Starbucks was not sustainable. But it seemed to work for some people. "The people happy there are in school and live with their parents. [Starbucks] were not really willing to work with people who wanted more—I mentioned it to my manager a few times, but she didn't do anything about it."

Of course, not all Starbucks employees were young people. "There were people with kids. Some had partners who helped them survive. But some were on food stamps and government assistance."

When Seattle city government passed a paid-sick-days ordinance, Starbucks management passed out flyers to Autumn and her co-workers informing them of their right to paid sick days. As is often the case in such settings, Autumn observed a difference between policy and practice. "If you were sick, you could call in and not be fired, but you were still responsible for finding someone to cover your shift. It was understood that you were expected to come in until they could figure it out. They'd say, 'You think you could come in for a couple of hours?' And then they'd try and ask you to cover the whole shift." As for the policy of paying employees when they asserted their rights and did not come in? "I never got a paycheck so I could never really be sure. They just didn't seem to follow the [new] law very well."

A Voice of Dissent

Autumn's greatest challenge at Starbucks came after she spoke up to try to better the situation. She became active with ROC and the Seattle-area Fight for $15. Soon thereafter, she was connected to a reporter from the *Seattle Times,* who interviewed her about her advocacy and took a photo of Autumn in her work uniform. "I thought it would be a small story," Autumn says now. "But I ended up on the cover of the *Seattle Times.*" The story, which ran in April 2014, focused on the plight of tipped workers across Seattle as a case for a $15 minimum wage.

Autumn didn't seek any additional attention, but it found her. "I didn't really care that much—and I didn't bring it up at work. But after that it seemed like corporate was keeping an eye on me." Autumn began to receive write-ups from her manager for work behaviors that had not previously been deemed problematic.

"I was getting written up for things like 'failing to comply with the barista job description,' which says we should always be smiling."

Autumn also reports receiving decreasing hours in the weeks and months after the newspaper article. "At first I was getting 22 hours; after the Seattle Times, I started getting 15 to 16 hours."

Shortly after the *Seattle Times* coverage, Autumn came face to face with Howard Schultz while working a shift. The cult of personality that surrounds the CEO—stories in employee literature about how or why he did this or that, first-person announcements in Schultz's voice, personal statements from the man in charge to his hundreds of thousands of employees—gave Autumn pause. So too did the recent media coverage, which she was sure Schultz had seen. Still, "He didn't say much to me; I made his latte. He was quiet."

Ultimately, when Autumn just could not survive on the hours she was getting, she decided to leave Starbucks. Far from being a place where debate and dissent was encouraged, Autumn felt pushed out because she endeavored to make things better for herself and her fellow workers. She went to a different coffee shop—an independent store with a completely different culture. She remains positive about the work and the business. "I like being a barista. I would like to work at a nice coffee shop, where you learn to make real coffee."

Autumn knows many other workers like her at Starbucks who are truly interested in the craft of coffee making but who are reprimanded for not following the automated coffee process in a certain manual-dictated order. Again, far from the place of discussion and creativity that epitomized the original coffee house, Starbucks, in Autumn's mind, is the ultimate corporate machine. "I'm on online communities with thousands of other Starbucks employees, and I've found it's more or less the same everywhere. Everybody who works at Starbucks complains about not getting enough hours. They make fun of the ridiculous things, the recipes, the names of the drinks." In the end, Starbucks wasn't for Autumn. "I'd like to make real coffee."

THE HIGH ROAD: MANIFESTO CAFÉ

Hassan Rashid Del Campo Nicholas was born and raised in Los Angeles. "My mother was born in St. Louis and grew up some in

Rhode Island, but she spent her formative years in San Diego. On weekends in the high school years, she'd come to LA. She knew that this was a place she wanted to stay; it was the big city, there were things to do. LA was seen as the city of opportunity." It was in LA that Nicholas's parents met, his father a Brooklyn native and son of a Haitian immigrant.

Although Nicholas's father worked as a stockbroker, his mother was a technician for the telephone company. "She was one of the only ladies climbing poles to fix the lines," Nicholas says proudly. "At one point, she became an account executive, but she always preferred to do the jobs that were traditionally seen as male—like going into the manholes."

Nicholas's mother and father divorced when he was young, and later his mother lost her job due to an unwillingness to relocate away from Los Angeles. It was then that Nicholas's comfortable lifestyle changed dramatically.

"I had grown up going to private schools, eating out. I didn't think we were rich, but I felt comfortable. When my mom lost her job, everything turned around. My mom was looking at shelters for us live in. We moved out of our duplex, out of our neighborhood. We went on public benefits. I remember going to the grocery store with food stamps. The whole thing really humbled me, made me appreciative of little things. It taught me to be resilient."

Nicholas now looks back on those days with fondness. "The worst economic times were my happiest. My mom and I were really close. We found a lot of ways to enjoy life on limited means, learned to find pleasure in little things. Getting ice cream could make your whole week."

Growing up with limited means but in a positive, supportive environment shaped Nicholas's values for the better. "I learned the significance of your environment—how that can affect your psyche. My mom, no matter what, tried to have us in a decent environment." After that, Nicholas says, the happiness flowed naturally.

"Since my mom was transparent about our expectations, I wasn't upset if I couldn't get certain things. I found joy in other things. I learned to be resilient and resourceful."

Starting Enterprises

After attending West Los Angeles Community College, then later earning a bachelor's degree at Loyola Marymount University in Los Angeles, Nicholas began working jobs at nonprofit organizations— first at an arts education nonprofit, and then another nonprofit that worked with entrepreneurs in the food industry. "We would help personal chefs and caterers start their businesses. We also worked with street vendors. [The] majority of the businesses were food based."

Nicholas concedes that there's a difference between his early jobs around the food industry and other jobs that actually involved working with food: "I never worked in a restaurant. I had applied for jobs, but never heard back."

His leap to the restaurant industry came through a neighbor in his downtown LA apartment building. "I had a friend in the building who had a friend that had gone to culinary school and was interested in opening up a café. One day we were all sitting in the building's common area, eating fried chicken. It was only the third time I'd ever met her, but she reached out and said, 'Hassan, I'm interested in starting a café. I know you're really artistic and creative. I'd love for you to be one of my partners.'" Hassan agreed, in part because he'd always harbored an interest in starting a restaurant—but also, he says, "I'm the kind of person who always says yes, though I had no idea of what I was undertaking."

In creating a concept for the new business, Nicholas and Christina focused as much on the physical and workplace setting as they did their business model. As it had been earlier in his life, Nicholas's focus was the environment. "We were both creative people, and we both had imaginations that were running wild. We were all about the vision, imagining this café. We were focused on the name, the colors, what it would [be] like, how people would feel walking in."

The partners' concept for Manifesto Café was centered on a desire to bring healthy, affordable, fresh food to an underserved community. This approach drew them initially to the somewhat infamous Skid Row neighborhood, an area of downtown LA often associated with poverty and crime. A coffee shop and café in Skid Row would serve as both an oasis to the underserved residents of the area and a destination for those living outside the area who were drawn to the unique business and unique setting.

Nicholas used connections from his previous nonprofit work to secure a location, funding, and support for the new enterprise. Getting buy-in from businesses and organizations already operating in Skid Row was paramount to the partners: "We wanted to make sure we weren't intruding on their space. We got their support, and some gave us letters that we used to help get financing."

The Skid Row real estate deal later fell apart. "We had a location," Nicholas recalls. "But the landlord was shady. Another location [in Skid Row] didn't work out either." Because the loan that Manifesto received came with requirements for how quickly the money was to be spent, the partners had to scramble. As Nicholas puts it, "We were on the clock. We needed to use the money or we'd lose it."

The next location to present itself was in Northeast Los Angeles, a somewhat stark departure from Skid Row in terms of landscape. The northeastern location was more residential, but attracted Nicholas and Christina because of its mixed demographic and relative dearth of other food sources. "It's a neighborhood in transition,"

Nicholas says. "There aren't many [food] options. This area was pre-viously low income, with a history of crime.

"We said, 'let's try to make this work.'"

Taking the High Road

Manifesto Café opened in May 2014 and now carries a staff of seven employees. Carrying on its owners' original mission, Nicholas and Christina focus on the source and quality of the café's offerings in addition to the revenue it generated. "That's been one of our tenets—healthy food that's tasty. It's always been our design to work with local, socially conscious vendors." Coffee at Manifesto is sourced from majority women-owned co-ops in Guatemala. Pastry vendors procure their ingredients from locally farmed markets.

The sourcing of Manifesto's products is admirable, but not hugely rare: cafes across the country have taken similar, admirable measures to offer better products that feed into an overall culture of environmental sustainability.

What sets Manifesto apart is the owners' willingness to go a step further: to cultivate an environment of employee enrichment and sustainability. "We wanted [working at Manifesto] to be more than a job," Nicholas says. "We want it to be a career where [employees] develop themselves." Manifesto employees are invited to orienta-tion at ROC-LA (where Nicholas is also a leader in the alternative restaurant association, RAISE), which, in turn, allows them access to job training.

Within the café, employees are encouraged to experiment with the coffee and food menus, and they receive a commission from sales of drinks or menu items that they develop; the menu now consists of three to four employee-developed items at a time. "We're allowing our employees to take part in creating our legacy, to take the journey with us," Nicholas says. "And we're transparent that it's a journey."

Having prioritized employee wages, the Manifesto ownership team has made these measures sustainable by creating efficiencies in other areas of the business. "We are re-negotiating
our lease; we are making the utilities more efficient," Nicholas
says. The team has also not taken its eye off Skid Row, their
original target for the business location. "We're maintaining our
relationship there. We've done pop-up and catering in partnership with Our Skid Row. We've provided food from the café to
the Downtown Women's Center. A lot of people that knew of
our plans of doing this work in Skid Row, and have kept us in
the loop."

The Manifesto Café sees itself as the complete antithesis of
Starbucks. "We're trying to send a message that we're going beyond
being a coffee shop. We're not just a coffee shop, we're a place for
civic engagement. We're a space for community gathering. It's like
back in Roman days—the watering hole where people come to
manifest. It's a place where people are coming to brainstorm ideas,
coming as a gathering place."

"Our employees are creating the space with us. That's the environment we want to create."

NOTES

1. William H. Ukers, *All About Coffee*, 2nd ed. (New York, NY: The Tea and
   Coffee Trade Journal Company, 1935), 15–17.
2. Ibid., 52, 68.
3. Heinrich Eduard Jacob, *The Saga of Coffee, the Biography of an Economic
   Product*, (London: George Allen & Unwin, 1935), 194–196.
4. Stephen Winick, "Coffeehouses: Folk Music, Culture, and Counterculture,"
   Library of Congress, April 17, 2014, http://blogs.loc.gov/folklife/2014/04/
   coffeehouses-folk-music-culture-and-counterculture/.
5. Melissa Allison, "Suit alleges "retaliation" by Starbucks," Seattle Times,
   February 9, 2007, http://www.seattletimes.com/business/suit-alleges-
   retaliation-by-starbucks/.

6. Alain Sherter, "For Some Starbucks Workers, Job Leaves Bitter Taste." *CBSNews.* CBS Interactive, September 26, 2014, <http://www.cbsnews.com/news/for-some-starbucks-workers-job-leaves-bitter-taste/>.

7. Rachael Larimore, "The Starbucks Guide to World Domination," *Slate,* October 24, 2013, http://www.slate.com/articles/business/when_big_businesses_were_small/2013/10/starbucks_business_strategy_how_ceo_howard_schultz_conquered_the_world.html.

8. Arthur A.Thompson, and A. J. Strickland. "Starbucks Corporation Case," in: *Strategic Management: Concepts and Cases,* 11th ed. (Boston, MA: Irwin McGraw Hill, 1999). 377.

9. Ahmed Alsawafiri, "The Startup Story of Starbucks," *Startup Bahrain,* May 1, 2013, http://startupbahrain.com/online/the-startup-story-of-starbucks/.

10. "Company Information: Our Heritage." *Starbucks Coffee Company.* January 20, 2015. http://www.starbucks.com/about-us/company-information.

11. "Starbucks Company Profile." *Starbucks Coffee Company.* January 21, 2015, <http://globalassets.starbucks.com/assets/4286be0614af48 b6b f2e17ffcede5ab7.pdf>.

12. Thompson and Strickland. "Starbucks Corporation Case."

13. Kateri Drexler, *An Encyclopedia of Mavericks, Movers, and Shakers, Volume 1,* (Westport: Greenwood Press, 2007), 323.

14. Alsawafiri, , "The Startup Story of Starbucks."

15. "Company Information: Our Heritage." *Starbucks Coffee Company.*

16. "Howard Schultz – Biography – Activist," http://www.biography.com/people/howard-schultz-21166227#early-life-and-career, (accessed February 27, 2015).

17. Thompson and Strickland. "Starbucks Corporation Case."

18. Melissa Allison, "Starbucks Co-Founder Talks About Early Days, Launching Redhook and Seattle Weekly, Too." *Seattle Times,* March 9, 2008, <http://seattletimes.com/html/businesstechnology/2004269831_bowker09.html>.

19. "Starbucks Company Profile." *Starbucks Coffee Company..* January 21,2015,

20. "Starbucks." *Forbes..* July 9, 2015, <http://www.forbes.com/companies/starbucks/>.

21. Jim Ewel, "The Transformation Agenda," *Agile Marketing,* June 3, 2013, http://www.agilemarketing.net/transformation-agenda/.

22. "Starbucks Company Profile." *Starbucks Coffee Company>,* January 21, 2015.

23. "Starbucks Company Timeline." *Starbucks Coffee Company..* July 9, 2015. <http://globalassets.starbucks.com/assets/5deaa36b7f454011a8597 d271f552106.pdf>

24. Ibid.

25. Victor Luckerson,. "These Are All the Awesome Benefits Starbucks Baristas Get." *Time.* June 16, 2014. Februaary 17, 2015, <http://time.com/2885743/starbucks-benefits/>.

26. "Starbucks Company Timeline." *Starbucks Coffee Company.* January 21, 2015.

27. Laura Lorenzetti, "Starbucks to Provide Free College Tuition for Baristas." *Fortune,* June 16, 2014, n.p,, , <http://fortune.com/2014/06/16/starbucks-to-provide-free-college-tuition-for-baristas/> (accessed February 17, 2015).

28. Ibid.

29. "Starbucks Union | IWW Starbucks Workers Union." *Starbucks Union | IWW Starbucks Workers Union.* n.p., n.d.; <http://starbucksunion.org/> (accessed January 23, 2015).

30. "Come Together for Striking Starbucks Workers," Starbucks Union, Industrial Workers of the World, November 7, 2013. http://www.iww.org/content/come-together-striking-starbucks-workers.

31. Alain Sherter, "For Some Starbucks Workers, Job Leaves Bitter Taste." *CBSNews.* CBS Interactive, September 26, 2014; Web. February 13, 2015, http://www.cbsnews.com/news/for-some-starbucks-workers-job-leaves-bitter-taste/ (accessed February 13, 2015).

32. Starbucks Worker Union. *Low Wages and Grande Profits at Starbucks: Report Summary.* August 2014, Web, <http://starbucksunion.org/sites/default/files/Low%20Wages%20and%20Grande%20Profits%20at%20Starbucks%20SUMMARY%20-%20August%202014.pdf> (accessed February 8, 2015).

33. Sherter, "For Some Starbucks Workers, Job Leaves Bitter Taste."

34. Jodi Kantor, "Starbucks to Revise Policies to End Irregular Schedules for Its 130,000 Baristas." *New York Times,* August 14, 2014, <http://www.nytimes.com/2014/08/15/us/starbucks-to-revise-work-scheduling-policies.html?_r=0> (accessed February 12, 2015).

35. Jodi. Kantor, "Working Anything but 9 to 5." *New York Times.* August 12, 2014, http://www.nytimes.com/interactive/2014/08/13/us/starbucks-workers-scheduling-hours.html?_r=0 (accessed February 16, 2015).

36. Jodi Kantor, "Starbucks to Revise Policies to End Irregular Schedules for Its 130,000 Baristas." *The New York Times,* August 14, 2014, <http://www.nytimes.com/2014/08/15/us/starbucks-to-revise-work-scheduling-policies.html?_r=0> (accessed February 12, 2015).

37. Alexander C. Kaufman, "Starbucks Vows to Raise Wages for Workers by January." *The Huffington Post.* October 17, 2014, <http://www.huffington-post.com/2014/10/17/starbucks-pay-bump_n_6003172.html> (accessed February 16, 2015).

38. Paul Solman, "More Part-Time Workers Face Instability, Long Hours to Make Ends Meet," PBS NewsHour, Transcript, September 1, 2014. < http://

www.pbs.org/newshour/bb/part-time-workers-suffer-instability-long-hours-make-ends-meet/ >.

39. Melvin Backman,. "Starbucks Workers Get Raises, New Dress Code and a Snack." *CNNMoney.* Cable News Network, October 16, 2014, <http://money.cnn.com/2014/10/16/news/companies/starbucks-policy-changes-tattoo/> (accessed February 16, 2015).

40. Kaufman, "Starbucks Vows to Raise Wages for Workers By January"; Sherter, "For Some Starbucks Workers, Job Leaves Bitter Taste."

[8]

DINERS

Change Is Possible

The diner is one of America's oldest and most universally patronized types of restaurant. Sometimes referred to as "lunch counters" or "greasy spoons," they're an archetype of 20th century America, and were accordingly the flashpoint for countless events of social and cultural change over the last several decades. From the sit-ins at lunch counters in Woolworth's department stores, to serving as the favorite lunch spots of civil rights leaders planning the March on Washington in Washington, DC, to the uproar over racial discrimination in Denny's restaurants, diners have been at the center of social upheaval and transformation in America.

Unfortunately, this upheaval has not yet delivered transformation to workers in America's diners. National diner chains—some the largest employers of America's full-service restaurant workers–are also more likely to provide the lowest wages.[1] Servers at America's diners can generally expect to earn, including tips, somewhere near the national median wage for tipped workers (approximately $8.70 per hour), no paid sick days, and no other benefits.[2] Mostly women, servers at diners too often experience sexual harassment from customers, co-workers, and management.[3] Many of these employees are mothers relying on tips to support their families, a reality that deincentivizes reporting of harassment. The spare-looking Table 8.1 illustrates how diner chains generally fare on wages, benefits, and promotions practices.

Of course, diners do not intrinsically have to provide low wages and benefits. Several of our high-road employer partners fall into the family-style category and fare quite well on raises, benefits, and promotions. See Table 8.2.

THE LOW ROAD: DENNY'S

Denny's receives a negative rating in every category rated in this guide. That is not to say that Denny's is a terrible company that is all bad all the time. Rather, Denny's is an example of a company that faced a financial and organizational crisis (in the form of the largest racial discrimination suit in recent history), then re-invented itself in the aftermath of that crisis. Although its reformation was focused on the treatment of consumers, not its own employees, the company's reformation is one of the best examples of how demand for change can produce exactly that.

Denny's was founded by a man named Harold Butler in 1953 in Southern California. Originally calling his restaurant "Danny's Donuts," Butler sought to provide "serve the best cup of coffee; make the best doughnuts; give the best service; keep everything spotless; offer the best value; and stay open 24 hours a day."[4] From the very beginning, Butler had ambitions of grand expansion. He focused on opening locations near highways and hotels and hungry travelers. Denny's became a publicly traded company in 1966, and reached 1,000 stores by 1981.[5]

However, Denny's parent company, Flagstar, took a serious downturn in the late 1980s and early 1990s. Several of the other brands in the company were in a serious tailspin. Heading toward

Table 8.1 LOW-ROAD RESTAURANTS

	$10+ Wage for Non-Tipped Workers	Hourly Wage for Tipped Workers Exceeds Minimum	Paid Sick Days	Promotion Practices	Stars
Big Boy					
Bob Evans Restaurant					
Cracker Barrel					
Denny's					
Friendly's					
IHOP					
Perkins Restaurant					
Shoney's					
Sonny's Real Pit Bar-B-Q					
Steak N Shake					
Village Inn					
Waffle House					

Table 8.2 HIGH-ROAD RESTAURANTS

	Hourly Wage for Tipped Workers Exceeds Minimum	$10+ Wage for Non-Tipped Workers	Paid Sick Days	Promotion Practices	Stars
Florida Avenue Grill Washington, DC			🔑	←	★
Good Girl Dinette Los Angeles, CA	💵	💲		←	★★
Honey Bee Diner Glen Burnie, MD	💵			←	★
TiGeorges Chicken Los Angeles, CA	💵	💲		n/a	★

*No tipped employees.

bankruptcy, in the early 1990s the company was hit with the greatest crisis of its existence—class action lawsuits based on countless incidents of overt racial discrimination against black customers.[6]

Guy Saperstein is a California attorney who was the lead plaintiff's attorney in the Denny's cases. He described the chain of events that led to Denny's incredible transformation: "[The plaintiffs] had gone to a Denny's restaurant late one evening after a college-preparatory conference. The young students were all dressed impeccably in suits and business attire, but were forced to wait to be seated. They observed many other white parties being seated and served while they continued to wait for service. At one point, when they inquired about being served, they were told that they would have to prepay for their meal. One young woman inquired at several other tables about whether other customers were asked to prepay, and all said they were not. The students left after an hour of waiting and not being served, thoroughly humiliated."

Soon after Saperstein's firm filed the case for the group of young people of color, they were contacted by an East Coast law firm that had a very similar case. "We suddenly realized this could be a nationwide class action lawsuit," recalls Saperstein. Countless more incidents were being reported to attorneys all over the country. A young girl told her family that on her birthday she wanted to eat at Denny's, which offered a free meal with proof of date of birth. The family, in a celebratory mood, took the girl's baptismal certificate with her birthdate to the restaurant but were immediately treated with extremely hostility and rudeness. The server and then the manager made a loud and public scene in rejecting the girl's baptismal certificate, saying that it could not constitute proof of the girl's birthdate. The family left, completely embarrassed and humiliated.

More and more cases kept flooding in, and the amount of publicity the cases were getting also started to increase rapidly. "Of all the cases I've ever done," said Saperstein, "no case ever got public attention like this. It was surprising how much this resonated with the public." The Denny's lawsuit was ongoing fodder for late-night talk shows for months.

After twelve different law firms had joined Saperstein in coordinating hundreds of cases of discrimination against black customers at Denny's restaurants, Saperstein received a call from Tom Fister, an attorney at a Los Angeles law firm representing Denny's. "I remembered him—he had played basketball at USC, and I had followed him as an athlete," said Saperstein. Fister asked to come to Saperstein's Oakland office to meet, and he was bringing the CEO of Denny's.

Saperstein agreed to the meeting, pulling together the dozen lawyers from the dozen law firms working on the case, and they listened in a conference room to the Denny's CEO speak. After initial pleasantries, the CEO said something curious: "He said he was going to make all kinds of changes in the company, and in good faith, he was going to give $3 million to 'negro' charities."

At this, Saperstein raised a hand. "I've heard enough," he said. He ushered the twelve other plaintiffs' attorneys into his office, then asked them what they thought of the offer. Their response, according to Saperstein, was unanimous: "Every single one of them, even my partner, seemed to think it was a good deal, a fine start."

Saperstein was the dissenting vote, and recalls how he voiced it: "'Gentlemen,' I said, 'if Denny's wants to do charity, that's fine by me. But that has absolutely nothing to do with this lawsuit.'" Saperstein recalls returning to the conference room and telling the Denny's CEO, "I just checked, and your earnings went from $200 million one quarter to negative $23 million last quarter. You're getting banged up on national television. I'm going to need $20 million by tomorrow morning for our clients, not to settle the case—we're going to need a lot more than that—but just to show good faith to me."

Saperstein's fellow attorneys were not happy, and communicated as much to him. But the gesture worked. "When I got to the office at 9:30 the next morning," Saperstein said, "Tom Fister was sitting in the lobby. 'We got your $20 million,' he said."

Aiding the plaintiffs' case was a similar incident involving President Bill Clinton's Secret Service team that occurred in May 1993. In town as part of a visit by President Clinton to the U.S. naval academy in Maryland, and his Secret Service agents went to breakfast at Denny's. A group of Black Secret Service officers were not served breakfast, whereas their fellow white Secret Service officers were seated and served promptly.[7]

The Secret Service incident elevated the class-action lawsuit to a level where it attracted even more national attention. In the end, Denny's parent company settled the case for $54 million, with a tremendous additional amount of injunctive relief—or mandated policy change.[8] The company signed a 100-page consent decree detailing every aspect of their business operations with regard to serving customers equitably, from where they advertised to how they trained all employees in the company on service. There were two full-time monitors to ensure that Denny's complied with all mandates.

Saperstein maintains that he never had a case in which he saw a company settle and make changes so swiftly and so completely. What was it that made this situation so different? "It was a bigger case than any other—with all the national television attention, more and more plaintiffs kept coming forward. We had between 6,000 and 7,000 plaintiffs, way higher than any other case I had ever litigated."

Ultimately, though, it came down to business. "The case had captured the national imagination. It was unusual to get all three national networks talking about a case. People felt like, 'It's 1990.' They could not believe the raw racial injustice. It hit a responsive chord." Denny's was losing an incredible amount of business, particularly among people of color. "It's not like they had a monopoly. People could choose to go somewhere else." And people did, in very large numbers.

Ongoing Change at Denny's

Denny's response to claims of customer discrimination was as thorough as it was swift. Long after attorneys had moved on to other cases, the company was undergoing a massive transformation. Principal among these changes was the addition of a new CEO, Jim Adamson, who documented the company turnaround in his book, *The Denny's Story.* In the book Adamson describes himself as the "turnaround guy" charged with bringing the company back from the brink of crisis. He describes himself as someone who grew up in a racially diverse environment, stepping into a company that suffered from real racial biases.

The Denny's Story describes Denny's corporate transformation in matters of racial justice as they apply to the restaurant's customer base, franchisor population, and board. The book includes very little discussion of employees. Adamson describes how the company spent tremendous resources overhauling their customer-service training for every single employee and manager in every single store—an enormous and costly initiative—as well as overhauling their marketing department, their franchisor program, and much more. For customers and franchisors, the changes were extreme, and Adamson fully admits that they were forced upon the company. "We learned the language of inclusion because we were forced to learn it; and then we learned to walk our talk to survive," he writes. ". . . [I]t would take the focus and intentionality that came with the pressure—and yes, the shame—of a consent decree to really make us understand how easy it was for any company, even with the best intentions in the world, to end up creating a climate that allowed people to be treated in a way that was biased and unfair."[9] Adamson describes how, as a result of his efforts, Denny's moved to have people of color as more than a quarter of all franchise operators, a few board members, and several managers.

Interestingly, initial resistance within Denny's to change with regard to racial equity in serving their customers echoes many of the same deeply-held beliefs among restaurateurs, including Denny's today, about why they cannot change their employees' wage, benefits, and promotions structures. Adamson writes how the company had initially felt that change would be too difficult and too expensive. He writes about how company employees seriously resisted when he tried to have the company celebrate Martin Luther King, Jr.'s birthday as a holiday.

Despite these setbacks, Adamson pushed change hard within the company, and, as he writes, not only because they were legally mandated to make changes. "The United States is not all white and never was," Adamson writes. ". . . [A]s businesspeople, we understand that there's a lot of money out there, that if we're responsive and respectful and address people's real needs, we've got a much better shot at getting a larger share of those dollars."[10]

In other words, change at Denny's ultimately came down to one thing: consumer power. Consumers left Denny's when Denny's became the poster child for racial injustice, and Denny's did everything in its power to rectify that image, by actually changing its practices. It follows that consumer power could likewise move Denny's to do better by its workers as well. If consumers could be outraged by raw racial injustice in 1991, certainly consumers can be outraged by women, including millions of women of color—being paid $2.13 an hour and suffering from severe sexual harassment in 2015. Denny's claims to be the nation's largest family style restaurant chain, so if consumer power could change Denny's, that would change the standard for millions of workers in the other major family-style chains as well.

Working at Denny's

Denny's has not yet felt that pressure from consumers, or anyone else, on the matter of livable wages for its employees. As conversations about income inequality and the minimum wage rose to a feverish pitch in 2014, the current CEO of Denny's Jim Miller, was reported to have dismissed questions surrounding the poverty of his workforce. As Yahoo News reported:

> As for the argument that no one can feed a family earning minimum wage, Miller says that's an issue for the employees and their families to work out for themselves. Denny's pays slightly better than the free market rate for the work they offer. If that's not enough for a worker perhaps a job at Denny's isn't the right fit.[11]

At least one operator of forty Denny's locations joined several other restaurant companies in 2013 in announcing that it would reduce all its workers' hours to less than thirty in order to avoid having to pay into the Affordable Care Act exchanges.[12]

As detailed in Chapter 1, 70 percent of tipped workers in America are women, who largely work at restaurants like Denny's—businesses that pay an untenable wage and put the onus of their workers' susbsistence on consumer tipping.[13] With wages from their employer ranging from between $2.13 and $5 an hour, these women live almost exclusively off their tips, and accordingly face an incredibly precarious and unstable livelihood. Living off tips makes these women vulnerable to manifold social threats, including but not limited to sexual harassment.

It's telling, then, that in 1997, after all the customer discrimination lawsuits had been settled, Denny's was hit with several additional lawsuits that did not receive nearly the same attention as the first: lawsuits by workers, not customers. In one lawsuit, describing sexual harassment suffered at a Denny's in Maryland, women claimed they were "called demeaning and derogatory names, forced to adhere to a strict dress code that was not enforced for male workers, and humiliated in front of colleagues and customers." One waitress claims a male co-worker intentionally splattered hot grease on her and made a "crude, sexist comment." Another waitress claimed that two male co-workers locked her in a walk-in freezer.

Several waitresses claimed that they were subjected to "sexist remarks and blatant sexual comments" at work. The waitresses "also said they were repeatedly warned that they would be forced to wear pieces of burned toast around their necks in the restaurant if they failed to bring food to customers on trays. A piece of toast was hung in a Denny's office as a reminder of the policy, the suit says, and one waitress was allegedly ordered to wear toast around her neck during her shift."[14] In recent years, Denny's has settled any number of these sexual harassment lawsuits.

As these lawsuits alleging such ongoing violations indicate, Denny's has a long way to go to extend the tremendous transformation of its customer service, that Adamson was so proud of, to its own employees. However, the Denny's story remains a source of great hope. If such a large company can make such dramatic changes so rapidly because customer pressure demands that they do so, and if Denny's found a way to work racial equity for customers and franchisors into their business model when they previously argued that they could not afford to do so, certainly customer pressure can move Denny's to change its business model with regard to wages and working conditions. They could even take a look at the financial model of the Florida Avenue Grill, a stand-alone diner that manages to provide much higher wages and benefits while thriving.

THE HIGH ROAD: THE FLORIDA AVENUE GRILL

In 1944, Lacey C. Wilson, Sr. and his wife Bertha opened the Florida Avenue Grill in Washington, DC, with money Wilson had saved from tips he had received shining shoes on Capitol Hill. Wilson envisioned a place that would provide a refuge for his fellow African Americans who'd been rejected from other local establishments.

The restaurant consisted of nothing more than a counter, two stools, and a basement kitchen. Like most restaurants, the early days were a struggle. Profit margins were so slim that Lacey and Bertha Wilson would buy two chickens, fry them, sell them, and then use the income to buy two more chickens. It follows that the Grill is described as being built "two chickens at a time."

Over time, however, the Grill became a local institution. In the early 1960s, as the civil rights movement was forming, organizers met at the Grill to plan the historic March on Washington in 1964. As Bertha Wilson was later quoted by the *New York Times*, the Rev. Martin Luther King, Jr. was at the Grill for one such occasion.

In 1968, when Martin Luther King, Jr. was shot and the District was aflame with uprisings, the Florida Avenue Grill stood in the epicenter of the turbulence. Wilson stayed up all night with a shotgun at the first booth to protect his restaurant, at one point putting out a fire after the Grill itself was firebombed. The business was one of only a few to withstand the turmoil. Two years later, in 1970, the Wilsons' son, Lacey Jr., took over the business and expanded it, purchasing the building it was housed in and the parking lot behind it. The restaurant remained a neighborhood and city staple throughout the1970s and 1980s, decades of notorious strife in the DC metro area.

New Ownership, New Vision

Imar Hutchins tells the story of how his great-great grandfather, a slave in the 1840s named Dyer Johnson, successfully bought his own freedom. Johnson was a carpenter whose skills prompted his owner to "rent" him to neighboring slaveowners, allowing Johnson to keep a fraction of the rent for himself. After several years of saving money, Johnson told his owner that one of the renters had inquired about buying Johnson permanently. When Johnson's owner named a price—$1300—Johnson produced the money and said that the purchasing slaveowner would need a receipt. "Sure," said the slave-master. "Who should I make the receipt out to?" When Johnson gave the name "Dyer Johnson," the master obliged, and Johnson was free, later buying his wife and children out of slavery as well.

At the end of his life, Johnson left his family a log cabin and a plot of land. He told his children, "I leave you this house where you can live; on this land you can grow your own food; and most important I leave you your freedom. I lived in slavery—it's hell. I've pulled a wagon up the hill this far. You need to keep it from rolling back down. If you need to put a brick behind the wheel and stop, then do so. But don't ever let it roll backwards." As his great-great grandson Hutchins attests, "That story has been passed down in my family to each new generation."

Each generation of Hutchins's family followed the tradition of progress—trying to keep the wagon moving. Hutchins's grandfa-ther was very active in the civil rights movement, desegregating schools in Kentucky. In fact, his grandfather's was one of the cases that led to the *Brown v. Board of Education* Supreme Court case.

Hutchins's grandfather's activism had a great impact on his own thinking and life.

"Thus began a tradition of trying to move forward each generation," says Hutchins.

In 2005, Hutchins was a Morehouse- and Yale Law-educated entrepreneur and with a successful restaurant venture already under his belt. While an undergraduate at Morehouse, Hutchins was a founder of Atlanta's first raw, vegan restaurants, Delights of the Garden.

When Hutchins purchased the Florida Avenue Grill in 2005, they weren't actually interested in the restaurant; it was as part of their larger acquisition at Florida Avenue and 11th Street—by then a bustling area—where he sought to build a sleek, green condominium building on the Grill's parking lot. Out of respect for the Grill's incredible history, Hutchins and his partner named the building The Lacey, selling units for between $250,000 and $1,000,000 each.

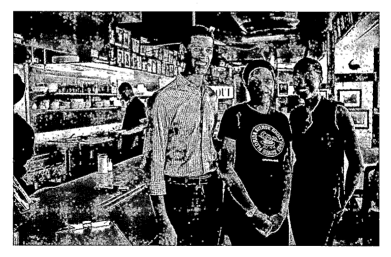

Imar Hutchins with Florida Avenue Grill staff.

After developing the building and garnering architectural praise for it, Hutchins sold the apartments in the Lacey—but kept the adjoining Grill. Hutchins's motives were largely preservational at the time: he knew that most other developers would be inclined to tear the landmark down.

Hutchins applied his family's spirit of progressivism to the restaurant beginning in 2012. He began by modifying the Grill's offerings while staying true to its legacy and fare—retaining its décor, homey feel, and soul-food concept but embracing concepts of health and sustainability in its business practices. Changes to the menu included the infusion of locally sourced ingredients and with additional vegetarian options.

Changes to how Florida Avenue Grill compensated its workers were intentionally less subtle. "I just did things based on feel," Hutchins says. "If you pontificate about it, you'll never do it. If you just say 'that seems fair,' then you'll just do it, and the world keeps spinning." Later, he increased the wages for his tipped workers as well.

To start, Hutchins allotted five paid sick days and five paid vacation days to each of the restaurant's fifteen to twenty employees each year. Next, he increased the starting wage for both tipped and nontipped workers to $9.50 per hour—"Really we were paying most people more, but we learned to pay attention to the starting wage as well."

These seemingly small changes in Hutchins' approach as an employer are part of his larger goal to effect cultural changes in how the restaurant industry lives—and how society regards the restaurant industry. "I want [working in a restaurant] to be viewed as a profession," he says. "It's such a misconception that people only work in restaurants when they can't do something else. Some people like it and want to do it because it coincides with who they are, but they have to fit into a system that's established. Service is something they see themselves doing long term.

"Fine dining servers are viewed as professionals, but I'd like to see it professionalized, period. Even in a place like mine. It should be like being a teacher or a police officer or firefighter. Service is what we do, and it's valued."

Hutchins has seen first-hand the sexual harassment and gender inequity that emerges from the lower minimum wage for tipped workers. "We need to change this system so that these women shouldn't have to wear tight clothes to do their job[s and] to get their tips. They should be able to make enough money to live with a modicum of comfort. That's what I'm trying to create."

As the Florida Avenue Grill continues to experience a booming business, Hutchins now faces questions of how to expand—the same ones that faced the Wilson family more than a half century ago. Hutchins' approach is unsurprisingly progressive: in cooperation with ROC, he is developing the second floor of the grill under a separate business imprint called COLORS on the Grill. Expanding on Wilson's vision for a place where elected officials can meet the restaurant workers they impact with legislation, COLORS on the Grill will also represent the tenets of sustainable fine dining and the economic empowerment of low-wage workers to the promotion of healthy environments and communities.

In all this, Hutchins is embracing the idea of a triple bottom line at the Florida Avenue Grill: measuring success in terms of social, environmental, and financial impact. "I'm trying to feed people's bodies and their minds. It was somewhere in my dharma to teach my people how to eat better. In the process, I'm not going to stop there, not going to divorce the food from the whole restaurant experience. We shouldn't be providing great food but treating people like crap. The day is going to come when even Zagat will have a fifth column—for workers."

NOTES

1. IBISWorld, Chain Restaurants Market Research Report, January 2015 http://www.ibisworld.com/industry/default.aspx?indid=1677, (accessed on Feb 24, 2015).
2. Restaurant Opportunities Centers United (ROC United), *Behind the Kitchen Door: A Multi-Site Study of the Restaurant Industry* (New York, NY: ROC United, 2011).
3. ROC United, Forward Together, et al. *The Glass Floor: Sexual Harassment in the Restaurant Industry* (New York, NY: ROC United, 2014).
4. "America's Greatest Brands: Denny's," *America's Greatest Brands*, 9, http://www.americasgreatestbrands.com/volume9/assets/AGB%20pdfs/AGB%20Dennys.pdf, (accessed 24 February 2015).
5. "History," *Dennys.com*, http://www.dennys.com/#/about/history (accessed 24 February 2015).
6. "Flagstar Companies, Inc." International Directory of Company Histories. 1995. *Encyclopedia.com*.http://www.encyclopedia.com/doc/1G2-2841400107.html (accessed February 24, 2015).
7. Michael A Fletcher, "Denny's settles bias suit," *The Baltimore Sun*, May 25, 1994. <http://articles.baltimoresun.com/1994-05-25/news/1994145038_1_ denny-restaurant-chain-secret-service-black-customers>
8. Stephen Labaton, "Denny's Restaurants to Pay $54 Million in Race Bias Suits," *New York Times*, May 25, 1994. http://www.nytimes.com/1994/05/25/us/denny-s-restaurants-to-pay-54-million-in-race-bias-suits.html.
9. Jim Adamson, *The Denny's Story: How a Company in Crisis Resurrected Its Good Name and Reputation* (New York, NY: Wiley, 2000), xiv, 18.
10. Ibid, p. 74.
11. Jeff Macke, "$15 Minimum Wage? Denny's CEO Weighs in on Worker Pay Battle," Yahoo! Finance, August 19, 2013, http://finance.yahoo.com/blogs/breakout/15-minimum-wage-denny-ceo-weighs-worker-pay-162034442.html.
12. James Nye, "Denny's to Charge 5% 'Obamacare Surcharge' and Cut Employee Hours to Deal with Cost of Legislation." *Mail Online*. November 15, 2012. <http://www.dailymail.co.uk/news/article-2233221/Dennys-charge-5-Obamacare-surcharge-cut-employee-hours-deal-cost-legislation.html>,(accessed Feb. 27, 2015).
13. ROC United, Family Values @ Work, et al., *Tipped Over the Edge: Gender Inequity in the Restaurant Industry* (New York, NY: ROC United, 2012).
14. Scott Higham, "Workers Accuse Denny's of Bias Waitresses Say Chain Allowed Harassment at Outlet in Edgewood." *Baltimore Sun*. n.p., June 27, 1997, http://articles.baltimoresun.com/1997-06-27/news/1997178052_1_ waitresses-harassment-denny (accessed February 27, 2015).

[9]

CONCLUSION

THE ROAD FROM HERE

The high-road restaurant practices described in this book are not always easy. Because nothing about owning or operating a restaurant is ever easy.

We at ROC have a lot of first-hand experience with the challenges of owning a restaurant. After ROC was founded in the months after the September 11, 2001 tragedy, my co-founder Fekkak Mamdouh and his fellow survivors from Windows on the World, the restaurant at the top of the World Trade Center shared a big idea: they wanted to open a restaurant together. They said it had always been a dream they talked about while at Windows, and now that Windows was gone, they wanted to work to make their dream a reality.

I was not interested in opening a restaurant; I told the workers that our mission was to improve wages and working conditions in the industry, not expand the industry. I was finally convinced by the promise of the business model they described: the restaurant would serve as a model of livable wages and working conditions, and could also house our training programs to help low-wage workers advance to livable-wage, fine dining service jobs in the industry.

Over the three challenging years that followed, I worked with ROC colleagues to develop the concept, design, and structure of the restaurant, identify the location, hire management, and raise the

$2.5 million necessary to open the restaurant in Manhattan. After several setbacks—including a particularly painful episode in which a small subset of the workers protested us, demanding all the not-yet-existent profits of the restaurant for themselves—we finally opened COLORS Restaurant in Greenwich Village in January 2006.

The COLORS restaurant—founded by World Trade Center survivors five years after 9/11, outfitted in décor by master designers and architects, with a menu of progressive and high-end fare—received so much media attention and fanfare that reservations were hard to come by in the first few months of opening. The buzz quickly died, however, as the quality of service was not able to meet the overwhelming demand. COLORS went through many months of financial hardships. The workers voted unanimously to reduce their pay—though still above average—until business picked up again. It did not sufficiently rebound, and in early 2007, COLORS received an eviction notice.

Over the next several years, we devised a series of schemes to keep COLORS open, and allow us to continue to pay above-average wages and provide benefits like paid sick days. We grew our private party business, holding a wide variety of functions and events in the restaurant. We expanded the training programs in the restaurant to serve hundreds of workers. Having found some amount of stability, we opened a second COLORS Restaurant in Detroit in 2010. By implementing all our lessons learned in New York, and with a much lower rental price, COLORS Detroit turned out to be far more manageable than COLORS New York. Nevertheless, our greatest challenge in both places remained constant throughout: we struggled year after year to find managers who both knew restaurant management well enough to help us crawl out of an ever-growing hole *and* were committed enough to the principles of high-road business practice that the restaurant advanced without hurting the mission. We, of course, got to know many successful restaurant owners and managers over the years who were joining our growing high-road restaurant group, RAISE, but we could not lure any of them away to work with us on COLORS. Most restaurant managers whom we were able to recruit had been trained in the traditional way of doing business: if the restaurant is not doing well, cut labor costs first.

Our miracle happened in the form of Rosanne Martino.

ROSANNE THE RESTAURANT MANAGER

Rosanne Martino grew up in the Sunset Park neighborhood of Brooklyn, New York. After her father died, Martino worked simultaneous jobs in a variety of industries to help support her mother: retail, finance, garment manufacturing, theater, and, naturally restaurants.

Martino's first job in the fine-dining sector was at the Greenwich Village institution One if by Land, Two if by Sea, where she worked doing comptroller work beginning in 1993. The restaurant, well known in New York for its eighteenth-century architecture and ambiance, had all the antiquated workplace trappings of an establishment that had been in business since the early 1970s. As Martino recalls the employee treatment upon her arrival, "It shocked me. The management at that time was only paying health insurance for managers. Workers would have to pay for having broken a glass. Pregnant women were only in the kitchen, as pastry cooks. If someone got pregnant, they'd say, 'she's out!'"

Martino's legacy at One if by Land would be defined by prevailing upon the owners to let her uproot these old-guard practices in favor of more progressive ones: the company hired servers of both sexes and all ethnic backgrounds, promoted from within, and offered employees livable wages, health care, paid sick days, vacation, and even a 401k.

Getting Involved with Changing the Industry

Martino and ROC first came in contact in the early 2000s, when we assembled high-road restaurant owners in the New York area in meetings that became known as the "Restaurant Roundtable." It was immediately evident that her values aligned with the organization's values. Even though Martino had instituted changes at One if by Land by more or less following her personal values, the roundtable network was able to fill in knowledge gaps in other areas. I never knew you have to pay extra when people work ten hour days, or that 'shift pay' is illegal," Martino recalls. "It was great to have someone tell you, 'This is the law.'"

"It was great to be told how to do it right, because I wanted to do it right, in a nonjudgmental situation. There were other restaurants in New York doing it right, who were very willing to share their successes, and what made it work for them. How they were able to pay people and still survive."

The consensus among restaurants participating in the Restaurant Roundtable was that it's possible to invest in workers and still make a profit by creating efficiencies in other areas. "There's always waste to be cut," Martino says. "Like burning fewer candles. If you're tighter on things that are less significant, the savings add up." With the dozens of local restaurants represented at the meetings, these efficiencies were extended to health benefits, too: "We talked about doing it as a collective, as a group, to reduce the costs," Martino says. "The ideas were great. There were lots of starts and stops, but over the years we have become much stronger, with some really good people involved."

In the eight years that followed, Martino emerged as a leader within the Roundtable and an ambassador for ROC's mission. In 2013, when ROC's job-training program for women, people of color, and immigrants (called CHOW, or COLORS Hospitality Opportunities for Workers) was temporarily displaced by renovations to COLORS' New York location, Martino was approached about hosting the training programs at One if by Land.

The timing of the request wasn't ideal: One if by Land had just hired a new, young, Cordon Bleu-trained chef named Colt Taylor, a rising star in the culinary industry who'd been brought up in the old way—by chefs who believed that you had to be maniacal to be a real chef. A similar old-guard approach had been demonstrated by Taylor's predecessor and had resulted in a lawsuit by employees against the restaurant in 1999. But Taylor was responsive to changing his approach and, in fact, became a leader in both compassion and the high road.

The ROC collaboration represented a potential new direction for the restaurant and its executive chef—one that they ultimately embraced. In addition to hosting classes for CHOW, Taylor and One if by Land became a signpost for the new way. Taylor summarized his (and his restaurant's) new approach in an op-ed published by the *Huffington Post*:

> Being compassionate isn't the same as being weak. Sending a sick employee home and paying them for the day doesn't breed laziness. Finding people's potential and patiently teaching them engenders loyalty. Compensating people fairly for their work doesn't make a restaurant unprofitable ... Abuses are no longer acceptable, and it is important to create a comfortable work environment, acknowledge workers' lives outside the restaurant, and provide decent wages and benefits.

The CHOW training courses at One if by Land were a benefit to both the trainees and the employees who trained them. As Martino recalls, "They would mix in with our staff, and our staff was really proud that we were doing it." Several of the students later found permanent jobs at One if by Land.

As One if by Land served as an outpost for ROC career training, the Restaurant Roundtable continued to grow in membership and momentum. Seeking to capitalize on this, the roundtable transitioned from a local high-road employers' group into an alternative national restaurant association called RAISE (Restaurants Advancing Industry Standards in Employment), one that aims to effect larger change through advocacy and leading by example.

Working on behalf of RAISE and its causes, Martino tells the story of a 2014 meeting between RAISE and a U.S. Senator in Washington. "We went into the Senator's office and were treated so poorly. The staffperson said, 'We have no room for you, we'll have to go meet over here.' It was a tiny room, like a closet. It was weird because everyone else had been so nice to us. When we finally sat down, [the staffperson] said, 'Ok, I don't have more than five minutes, what's your story?' So the employers started talking. After just a few seconds the staffperson says, "Wait!! You guys are from ROC? I thought you were from the NRA. That's why I was treating you like shit! They always say the same things.' We said, 'So you don't really only have five minutes?' He said, 'Hell no! I have time. Please talk to me. Please tell me your stories.' To me that showed that things have really changed."

Martino and sixteen other high-road employers from all over the country—including Paul Saginaw of Zingerman's—worked to create a vision for RAISE. Saginaw led the session, Martino recalled. "When we went into the room, we were visioning with Paul, it was amazing to see how far this could go. We were all throwing out a million ideas, and I thought, 'This is really great!' I came back, bubbling over with the news. Colt and I and even the other employers were really excited with the possibilities."

Taking Over COLORS

Martino and Taylor started talking more with ROC Co-Director Fekkak Mamdouh. "We wanted to know why COLORS was still under renovation. Mamdouh told us that ROC was looking for a partner to help turn the restaurant around. He said, 'You guys want to do it? Let's walk over there.' When we went there, we were amazed—the space, the kitchen, everything was working."

Martino and Taylor got excited by the possibilities, and at some point their excitement conflicted with their role at One if by Land. "At One if by Land, as much as Colt and I had a lot of say, there were other things we wanted to do. When we got involved with ROC & CHOW, Oscar was like, 'Why are we doing this, are we One if by Land or something else?' When it came to hiring, we wanted to give people a chance, but there was some resistance. We said, 'Wouldn't it be nice if we could really hire the people we want from CHOW, go 100 percent into this? That's what spurred us on. For Colt it was also the idea that he'd have the freedom to experiment in the kitchen. For me, it was the thinking that we can really help people, without any owner to say, 'She looks a little funny.' It was a perfect marriage of what we were trying to do at One if by Land but couldn't do because there were other people who had other ideas."

Martino and Taylor decided to enter into a full partnership with ROC to completely overhaul the decor, menu, and service at COLORS Restaurant. It became a labor of love. "First of all, all the CHOW students got involved in everything. The staff at One if by Land came to help—even the plumber—because they believed in the project. We spent the whole summer working, wanting to get it open. Everyone couldn't wait to work there. That was really great."

Taylor had an exciting idea for the menu; through lots of experimentation he had devised a way to cook almost everything completely gluten free. "The customers started coming in. My daughter is a celiac, and she will travel anywhere in the world to eat good gluten free food. For gluten free folks, there's always certain food they'll feed you—risotto. You don't get fish and chips; you don't get fried chicken. That was the goal—to be able to have a piece of cake, a piece of bread, that doesn't taste like cardboard. With Colt's menu, people don't even have to know it's gluten free. We have a raspberry chocolate ganache with coconut whip cream that you'd never know was vegan and gluten free. Gluten free folks always feel like oddballs when they go out to eat; here there's something for everyone, and you don't have to go off your special diet. It was a gamechanger."

ROC United board member Jennifer Herman owned a construction company and donated a complete renovation of the restaurant; customers were wowed with the new look. ROC members who had gone through CHOW would work at the newly renovated restaurant for a short period of time and then move on to work at other fine dining restaurants. "People who started here would start coming back like the older brother or sister, to say, 'He should be serving it this way.'"

Martino eventually left One if by Land to join ROC's staff as our national COLORS project manager, helping to manage COLORS Restaurants in New York and Detroit, and helping to open new COLORS restaurants in Washington, DC, New Orleans, and Oakland, California. What excites her the most, however, is the people she came to know who have been through the program and the restaurant, and who've managed to turn their lives around.

"Lamont went through CHOW and was hired at One if by Land. One day he came into the coatcheck room and told me, 'I have to tell you something. I was really hopeless. After my first orientation into CHOW, I came home and told my mother, 'I think this could change my life.' I don't have to run the streets anymore. I'm going to be the one in my family to turn this family around.' His family is counting on that. You don't know the desperation and hopelessness in people's lives in some neighorboods where they don't see an example of anything different. He's doing well, he has people who believe in him, teaching him. He's building [a] career for himself, to support himself."

"Ceb went through CHOW. He had a military background, and he couldn't hold onto a job. He worked for a while at COLORS, and then I sent him over to One if by Land to work when they told me they needed extra people for a brunch. The waiters are really tough at One if by Land, but everyone said, 'This guy's a superstar,' and they asked him back to work there. He's really good."

Martino is especially proud of the women: Marilyn, with five children, producing amazing gluten-free pastries; Dominique, who chose a profession in hospitality and is quickly moving up the ranks; Meena, who was inspired to wear her hair naturally—rare for New York City servers of color—by Dominique.

After nearly a decade of struggle, COLORS—the restaurant owned by the worker movement—has turned around under Martino's leadership. The restaurant was named one of the top-ten restaurants to visit on Thanksgiving and was also named the top gluten-free restaurant in New York City. Most importantly, the restaurant is full. "I really like to help people. I'd love to see this restaurant be really successful. I'm not creative in any other way—I don't draw or paint or sing. What I can do is look at other people's visions and try to make that happen. My contribution is to help other people's creativity. That gives me a lot of sense of fulfillment. A lot of it is where your head is." When Martino first came to COLORS from One if by Land, she struggled. "It was godawful. It was freezing, the pipes kept breaking, and it was creepy at night.

One night after everybody left, I locked the door, looked around, and spoke to the room. I said, 'It's not creepy, there's good energy here. I started liking the energy, loving the space. I said aloud, 'I love this space.' Like I used to love One if by Land. I don't know what it was, but like a miracle, people started filling the space the next day. You have to believe in it and it will happen."

Martino also has a special dream about COLORS NY. "I'd love this to be the place that restaurant workers come to late at night. Sardi's does an actor's menu with a difference price for actors. We're planning to do a restaurant workers' menu, where you'd only know about the restaurant workers' menu if you're a restaurant [worker]. I want it to be the place restaurant workers will hang out."

Martino thinks about her current work as a way to fix the disparities of the past. "It amazes me to think that when I talk about women not being able to work in Manhattan fine dining restaurants, I'm not talking about having come up in the business in 1910. I'm talking about the late 1970s and 1980s and 1990s, when there weren't opportunities for women in restaurants, in any kind of career that would be financially sustainable. Even to this day, in most places, I would not be paid what a man would be paid. There's still definitely a pay disparity that has to be eliminated. There's still a ways to go. It's great to be part of an organization that's actually actively making changes on a lot of different fronts."

After nearly twenty years of restaurant and management experience, how did Martino find this very unique path in the restaurant industry? "When I think about it, I really do feel like my maternal grandmother was the biggest influence in my life. She told me, with every new group that comes in, they get oppressed, and then they move up and they forget and oppress the next people. Stepping on people is not the way to move up. It's against logic in a way. Everyone thinks you just follow the past but that goes against logic. It's important to follow your own path."

The Future Of Our Forks

A restaurant's worth is largely measured by what critics say about it. Publications like Zagat's, Michelin Guide, and *New York Times* may differ in their subjects or tone, but they all evaluate based on the same basic criteria: food, service, ambiance, value.

Our food-fetishizing culture has taken restaurant criticism a step further by emphasizing the importance of food sourcing as a measure of the restaurant's overall quality. More and more, chefs today are careful to describe to customers how their food came to be on their plates—sustainably, locally, organically, biodynamically—as part of an overall understanding that better food practices contribute to a better world.

What's hidden in plain sight as we talk and talk about food is the glaring mistreatment of people whose work makes restaurants such an integral part of the U.S. culture and economy. Fair pay for the people who prepare and serve us our meals is the final frontier for the food service industry—and for a society that loves eating out.

The U.S. restaurant industry is at a fork in the road, and has to decide which path it will take. Will it take the path of the past, the path of poverty and oppression, of inequality and harassment, a totally unsustainable path for almost everyone who touches it? Or will it take the path of Martino and of so many other great restaurant employers profiled in this book and across America? The high road means livable wages and benefits that allow workers to stay home when they are sick and to see a doctor when they need to. The high road means allowing restaurant workers to advance up a career ladder and think creatively, as other professionals do, to innovate and experiment in ways that benefit everyone—workers, employers, and consumers. Most of all, it means a better industry for all—professional workers who are proud to provide quality food and service; responsible employers who enjoy healthy profits by enjoying highly productive workers who develop their craft by staying in one job for a long period of time; and well-fed consumers who experience healthy, safe, and delicious meals served by happier workers.

In fact, this is not just a fork in the road for restaurants; it's a fork in the road for our economy and for this country. We have a choice as a nation—we can continue down our current trajectory, and observe what abnormally high levels of inequality can do to our nation, how it devalues who we are as a country. Or we can follow the examples of the smart, profitable, and caring employers in this book and create an industry, an economy, and a nation that works for all of us.

As a nation, the fork in the road is also about the very nature of our democracy. Fundamentally, it comes down to one question: will we allow corporate trade lobbies like the National Restaurant Association to control our democracy, extend the legacies of slavery, and set the floor for wage and benefit standards in this country? Or should those decisions reside with the people and the representatives we democratically elect?

The restaurant industry is not the only sector of our economy that presents us with these choices, but it certainly offers a good place to start. The grave disparities between multinational restaurant corporations and their employees, the inequities faced by women and people of color, and the ways in which the industry forces consumers to pay their own workers' wages for them— epitomizes the fork in the road that the United States faces. Here's hoping we follow the path created by the extraordinary heroines and heroes profiled in this book, and the millions of workers in this industry who know that following the high road will benefit us all.

INDEX